Walking Will Save Your Life!

Walking Will Give You a New Life!

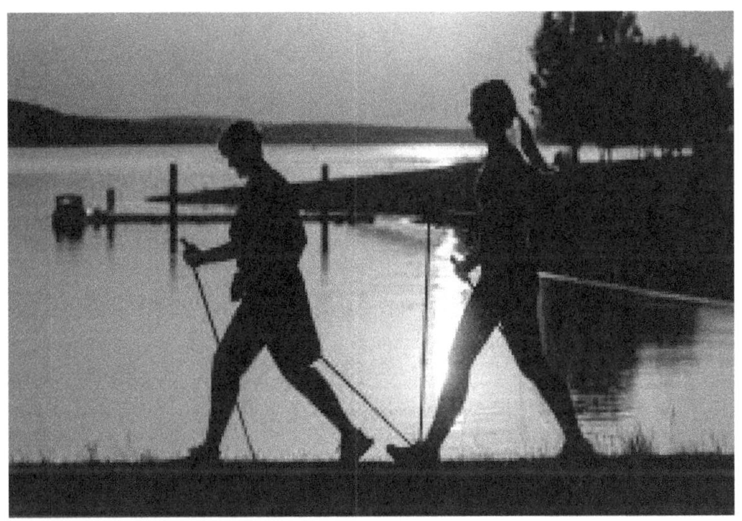

Allen Kelley

Allen Kelley

Walking Will Save Your Life

Walking Will Give You a New Life

Dedication

If you feel that there is something missing in your life, this is for you. Here is how to enjoy the greatest journey in the world!

Have you been searching for a simple way to improve your health, boost your mood, and extend your lifespan? The answer is as easy as putting one foot in front of the other. In the following pages, you will discover the incredible and scientifically proven benefits of walking and how this basic human activity can transform your physical, mental, and emotional wellbeing. Whether you're looking to lose weight, reduce stress, strengthen your heart, or just feel your best, walking could be the key to unlocking a healthier, happier you. Get ready to learn how walking will save your life – and give you a new life!

Table of Contents

Prelude

How A Daily Walking Regimen Saved My Life – and Gave Me a New Life!

A devastating motorcycle accident left me unable to walk. After several major operations, a surgeon sadly informed me that I would spend the rest of my life in a wheelchair.

Not a very good prognosis for someone who was a mountain climber, marathoner, triathlete, and avid hiker for most of his adult life.

I was not ready to give up! It was time to fight back!

I was working and living in Cottonwood, AZ at the time. I was aware of a hiking/walking trail that ran along the Verde River. The name of the trail was "The Jail Trail" as it started at a building that was a jail in the western cowboy days.

I checked out the beginning of the trail. It looked challenging - but promising for what I had in mind.

I was determined to master this fascinating piece of terrain and learn how to walk again!

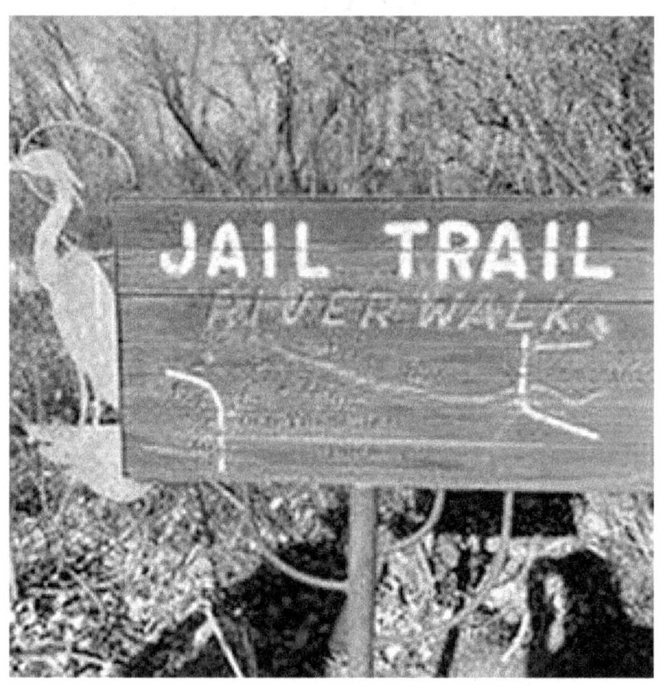

The following day I showed up early in the morning. I would see how far I could walk along the path without falling. I made it out a few hundred feet, and yes, I fell down a few times.

I came back the following day determined to walk farther without falling. I did manage to go further and fell once.

Progress, not perfection!

I continued to walk a little further every day and didn't fall most days.

After several months, I could navigate the trail to the end, and return to the starting point , without falling.

The day that I finally made the sojourn from beginning to end without falling was one of the best days of my life. I realized the greatest possible sense of accomplishment.

The best part of this whole adventure was this. I learned how to walk once again – something I had taken for granted.

I felt better than I had ever felt, and I attributed that great feeling and sense of accomplishment to my daily walking regimen.

No matter where you are at in your life with respect to exercise and specifically walking, don't deny yourself the gift of feeling great. To realize all the great benefits offered to you, read on.

Introduction

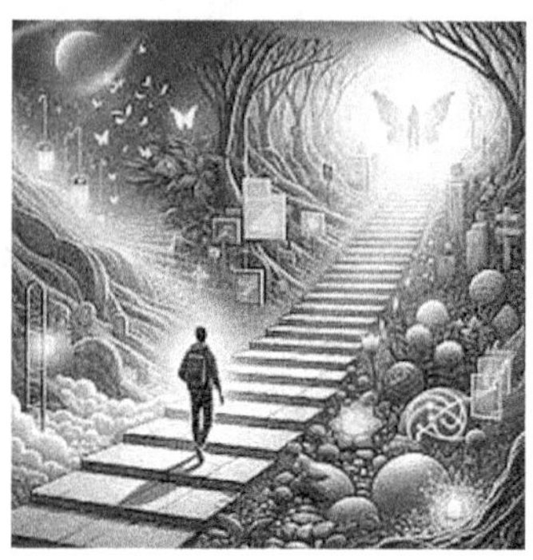

Welcome to the transformative world of walking! In these pages, we embark on a journey that goes way beyond mere steps. We delve into the profound impact walking can have on our physical health, mental well-being, and overall quality of life. Each chapter is a pathway to discovering the joys and benefits of putting one foot in front of the other, from the simple pleasures of movement to the profound insights gained along the way.

"Discovering the Joy of Movement" presented here invites you to reconnect with the innate pleasure of walking. Walking will you're your life delves into the scientific benefits that come with every stride. In "Exploring the Mindful

Walk," we embrace the meditative power of each step, learning to be fully present in the moment.

Life's challenges are met head-on in "Walking Through Life's Challenges," where the rhythm of walking becomes a steady companion through adversity. "Finding Inspiration in Every Step" reminds us that every journey, no matter how small, is filled with opportunities for growth and inspiration.

As you move through these pages, you will find that "Walking Toward a Better Future" explores how walking can be a catalyst for positive change, not just for us, but for our communities as well. "The Community of Walkers" celebrates the camaraderie and shared passion that comes from walking together.

"Walking as a Way of Life" goes beyond a mere activity, showcasing how walking can permeate every aspect of our daily routines. Whether it's walking for self-discovery, or walking to lose weight, walking to find yourself, or the transformative journey of walking, we uncover the profound impact that this simple, yet powerful act can have on our lives.

Join me as we step into the world of walking—a journey of physical vitality, mental clarity, and soulful exploration.

The Eric Pupek Story

"I Weighed 500 lbs. Walking Every Day Changed My Life"

By Eric Pupek

It was 2020 and, for some of us, the worst year of our lives. But, as the song goes: "Sometimes, darkness can show you the light".

With all that unfolded around us during the COVID pandemic, I found myself at 500lbs and with a job that had me traveling from home to hotels to hospitals, even though most of the world was shut down.

I had been overweight from a young age. In fact, I can't remember a time when I wasn't. But this was the largest I had ever been. I wore a 6XL shirt—I'm large and tall, so it was more like a 7XL because they always ran big—and had a 64-inch waist.

When I was home, I was stuck in my office, frustrated, scared, and uncertain of what was next. I lost several friends to COVID, and working in hospitals fueled everything that was going on in my head.

Was I next? Would I infect my family? I was frightened!

My wife urged us to go for a walk, suggesting that we stay away from other people and head into the woods. That is when I realized how out of shape I was.

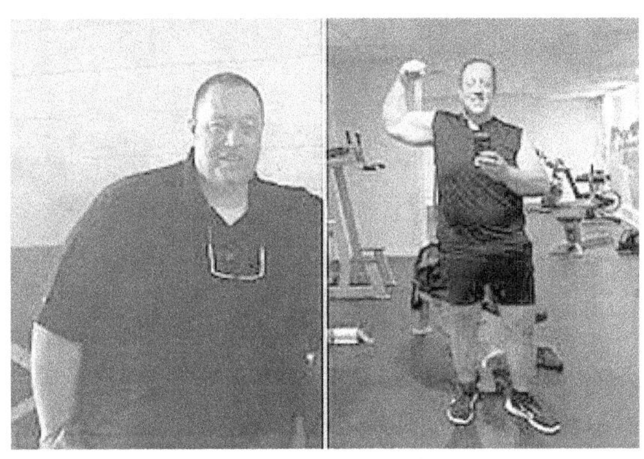

Eric Pupek pictured left, before his weight loss, and right, after. He started off weighing 500lbs before he began walking for exercise every day.

We walked a block: I was out of breath, my back and feet hurt, and it was a struggle for me. My wife was in much better shape than me. We'd been married for 27 years at that point, and you get to know a person and what drives them.

My wife never allowed me to quit. Every day, she would ask: "You want to go for a walk?" If I said no, I'd feel like I let her down, so I never did.

Amazingly, before I knew it, I'd lost 75lbs. It's a drop in the bucket when you weigh 500lbs, and I'd lost weight before only to gain it back. The last time I gained weight back, so I made a promise: If I ever lost weight again, I would never gain it back.

I knew what I had to do, and walking was the thing that allowed me to lose weight. I am driven and competitive, and if you tell me I can't, I will prove otherwise. I'm sure my wife knows that too; she has helped me fuel that fire.

I started walking everywhere. The only time I used my car was when I had to drive to the next hotel or hospital for work.

The funny thing about walking is it allows you to clear your mind, and it highlights the beauty around us. When you drive, you focus on what is ahead. But when you walk, you can see everything.

Walking also allowed me to hold myself accountable with food. If I had a craving for a large steak and cheese extra greasy—I mean, what other way is there to have one?—I would walk a mile to the (healthy) sub place, enjoy my meal, and walk back and not feel guilty.

I called it accountability. There's nothing worse than trying to lose weight and having a craving, so I didn't ignore that craving, I fed it. But the accountability freed me from the remorse afterward that usually led to more eating. I'd earned it.

The only time I felt remorse was when I didn't walk, so I walked every day. I started with a block, then a mile, then two miles. And every day I would push myself further. The next thing I knew, it was 5km every day.

This led me to find new places to walk. I started walking in the woods, parks, trails. I even got an app to show me what was available no matter where I was. It was exciting; where will I discover next?

I used to laugh when people would say they went for a walk in the woods. I would say: "Why?" I get it now.

Perspective: that's a huge word for me and one that has changed the way I live and how I see the world. Until you put yourself in someone else's sneakers, you will never have the perspective on what makes them who they are and why they do the things they do.

I took a job with a small startup that gave me the opportunity to travel the world. It was then I realized I had to document my journey of weight loss and personal growth, so I started the "Walking the World" group on Facebook.

The goal was to use the Facebook group to drive me forward and hold myself accountable. People around me started to notice what I was doing, and their support only drove me more. "Hey, I saw you walking, keep it up, looking good....proud of you."

I traveled to the Netherlands and walked from one end of the country to the other, from Groningen to Amsterdam and Rotterdam. I did 45,000 steps walking in Amsterdam alone one night. What an amazing city Amsterdam is, especially at night.

Then I was off to Paris, France. I arrived at 9 a.m. but the hotel room wasn't ready, so I walked to the Eiffel Tower and had a French roast coffee and a chocolate croissant. Again, accountability through walking and no regret—it was amazing.

Walking back, I was able to catch Vice President Kamala Harris and her motorcade driving past me on her visit to the Institut Pasteur.

Next stop was Lyon in France and the Parc de la Tête d'or and the amazing waterfront. Lyon is a beautiful city. With COVID restrictions ending, locals had set up restaurants on boats in the waterways for open seating. It was amazing to see how other countries handled the COVID crisis.

Then I was in London, England when my first stop was Abbey Road. Music has always been a huge part of my life and I don't know if I could have accomplished any of this without it.

As I approached, I sang "All You Need Is Love," only to have other people join in.

The day I hit my ideal weight and was approved to have all the extra skin taken from my abdomen; I celebrated. I hiked the Wishbone Trail from Carver to Plymouth in Massachusetts; 13 miles of every terrain possible.

It was like when you watch the final group on the TV show Survivor as they look back at the journey they had just traveled. It gave me strength and clarity. It spoke to me and said: If you want something bad enough and you never give up, you will accomplish it.

I have walked across the U.S. and Canada and made a trip to Manchester, England.

I have put a map of the world on my office wall and every time I walk somewhere new, I put a pin in. Someday, I will fill that map.

I am often asked: How much weight did you lose and what is your weight now?

I have lost over 217lbs so far, but the journey is ongoing. Along with weight loss I am working to build muscle. When you lose that much weight you also lose muscle mass, so it's important to build that back as well. How much you weigh is important, but quality of life and the things you can do outweigh that number.

My doctor told me I have added 40lbs of muscle and that is not the norm, but my body type is not one of a small man. I am 6'1 with a 14 EEEE size shoe. At some point, it is less about the number and more about your health and all the things I can do now that I have never been able to do before.

Don't get me wrong: I still step on the scale. But the mirror and my doctor are better indicators of my progress now. This journey is ongoing and will be part of my everyday life. I moved to Philadelphia after living all my life south of Boston.

My new adopted home has welcomed me and the people in the city of brotherly love have been amazing. I have a granddaughter and a grandson on the way. Living here allows me to enjoy every moment with them. Having the stamina to keep up with them is glorious.

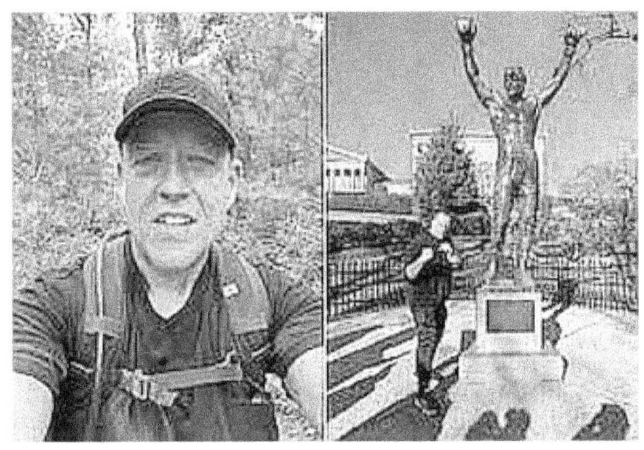

Eric Pupek at the Rocky Balboa statue in Philadelphia

My daughter is getting married this year. I was asked to be the officiant for her wedding, and I am working extra hard to look good, and I am going to dance the night away. There's always something new and exciting on this journey.

I have made it my goal to empower others to never give up. I am not an influencer, I am an empoweree. I will never tell you what is right for you, I will only tell you that if you want something bad enough: Yes, you can. It is never easy, and the journey may be long, but if you never give up: Yes, you can.

This journey did not happen overnight. You must start somewhere. I started walking a block and eventually hiked 13 miles, but I never quit and never gave up. I have a lot of people to thank for that.

All of you who honked your horns as I walked around town, and who encouraged me to keep moving—thank you.

A family friend who had not seen me in over a year almost rear-ended someone because he couldn't believe what he saw. Please keep your eyes on the road and thank you.

Now it's time for me to pay it back and that is why I wrote this. I want you to know, yes you can, just keep moving. Find your soundtrack and turn it up to 11 (Spinal Tap reference, FYI) because it's contagious.

I am proof of that.

Take a moment to listen to your soundtrack and that of the world around you. If you don't like what you hear, own it because only you can change it.

Eric Pupek is a husband, father and grandfather who changed his life one step at a time, walking the world.

Forward
Walking: The Secret Weapon

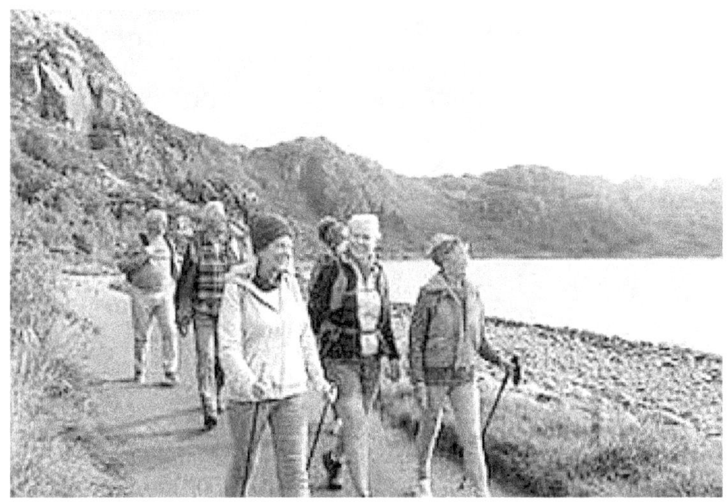

The Powerful Benefits of Walking

Here are brief descriptions of just a few of the exciting walking innovations and life altering concepts that will be covered in length in the following chapters. Enjoy ths exciting journey as you walk through this illuminating tome!

What if I told you there was a simple, free activity that could dramatically improve your physical health, mental wellbeing, creativity, longevity, and productivity? You'd probably be skeptical of such a bold claim. But the truth is, the "secret weapon" to a better life has been right under our noses - and feet - the whole time. That secret weapon is walking!

Walking is the unsung hero of exercise and an underrated superpower we all possess. It requires no expensive equipment, gym membership or training. Anyone can do it, just about anywhere, anytime. And a growing body of research shows that walking delivers an impressive array of health benefits.

In a world where people are constantly searching for the next big thing to improve their health and well-being, the answer may be simpler than we think. Walking is an activity that we often take for granted. It is a **secret weapo**n that can transform our lives in countless ways. In the following pages, we will explore the amazing benefits of walking and how it can be the super-power that empowers your life.

The Physical Benefits of Walking

Walking is a low-impact form of exercise that can provide a wide range of physical benefits. Regular walking can help you lose weight and maintain a healthy weight, reduce the risk of chronic diseases such as heart disease, diabetes, and certain cancers, and improve overall cardiovascular health. Walking can also help strengthen bones and muscles, improve balance and coordination, and boost immune function.

One of the most significant benefits of walking is its ability to improve cardiovascular health. Walking can help lower blood pressure, reduce the risk of heart attack and stroke, and improve circulation throughout the body. Studies have shown that walking for just 30 minutes a day can reduce the risk of heart disease significantly. .

Walking can also be an effective way to manage weight and prevent obesity. Walking burns calories and can help boost metabolism, making it easier to maintain a healthy weight. In addition, walking can help reduce the risk of type 2 diabetes by improving insulin sensitivity and glucose control.

The Mental Benefits of Walking:

Walking is not just good for the body; it can also have a profound impact on mental health and well-being. Regular walking can help reduce stress and anxiety, improve mood, and boost cognitive function.

One of the ways that walking can improve mental health is by reducing stress and anxiety. Walking can help clear the mind and provides a sense of calm and relaxation. It can also be a form of meditation, allowing individuals to focus on the present moment and let go of worries and concerns.

Walking can also be a powerful tool for boosting mood and combating depression. Walking has been shown to release endorphins, the body's natural mood-boosters. Regular walking can help improve self-esteem, reduce feelings of sadness and hopelessness, and promote a more positive outlook on life.

In addition to its emotional benefits, walking can also have a positive impact on cognitive function. Walking can help improve memory, attention, and decision-making skills. It can also reduce the risk of age-related cognitive decline and dementia.

The Social Benefits of Walking

Walking is not just a solitary activity; it can also be a social one. Walking with friends, family, or a walking group can provide a sense of connection and community that can be incredibly beneficial for overall well-being.

Walking with others can provide a sense of accountability and motivation to stick with a regular walking routine. It can also be a way to build and strengthen relationships, as walking provides an opportunity for conversation and shared experiences.

In addition, walking can be a way to explore new places and connect with the world around us. Walking through a park, a city street, or a nature trail can provide a sense of adventure and discovery that can be incredibly rewarding.

The Practical Benefits of Walking

Walking is not just good for our health and well-being; it can also be a practical and sustainable mode of transportation. Walking can help reduce traffic congestion, improve air quality, and save money on transportation costs.

Walking is a low-cost and accessible form of transportation that can be done anywhere, at any time. It requires no special equipment or training and can be easily incorporated into daily routines.

In addition, walking can be a way to explore and appreciate the world around us in ways that are not possible when driving or taking public transportation. Walking allows us to notice details and experience the world at a slower pace, providing a sense of connection and appreciation for our surroundings.

Walking is a 'secret weapon' that can transform our lives in countless ways. From improving physical health and reducing the risk of chronic diseases, to boosting mental well-being and providing a sense of connection and community, walking is a "super-power" that we all have access to.

So, the next time you are looking for a way to improve your health and well-being, consider lacing up your shoes and going for a walk. You may be surprised at just how powerful this simple activity can be.

Studies have found that walking for just 30 minutes a day can help you:

- Maintain a healthy weight and lose body fat
- Prevent or manage heart disease, high blood pressure and type 2 diabetes
- Strengthen your bones and muscles
- Improve your mood, cognition, memory, and sleep
- Increase your energy and stamina
- Enhance your creative thinking and problem-solving ability
- Reduce your risk of depression, dementia, and Alzheimer's disease

Those are some incredible advantages of an activity as simple as putting one foot in front of the other. Even a 10-minute walk can provide an immediate energy and mood boost. Walking is like a "wonder drug" - except there are no negative side effects, only positive ones.

Chapter One
The Joy of Walking

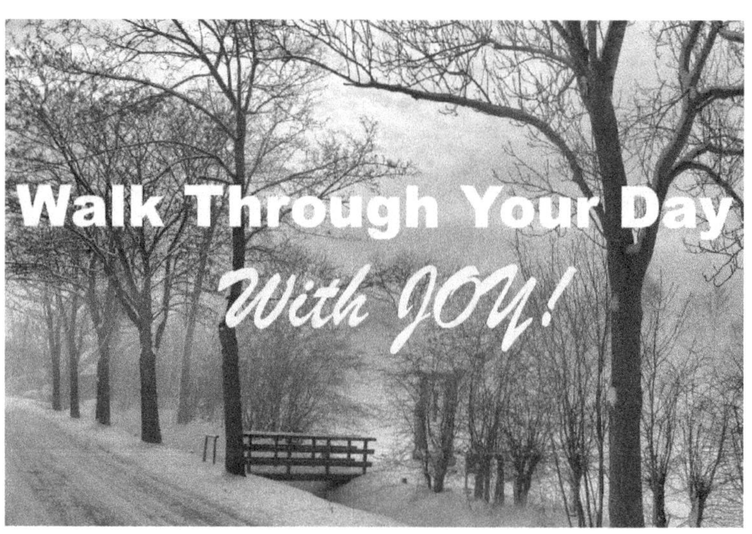

Walking is one of the most natural and joyful activities a person can engage in. There is a profound sense of freedom and connection that comes from propelling ourselves forward under our own power, one step at a time.

When we walk, we tune into the rhythms of our body and our environment in a way that is difficult to achieve through other forms of movement. The steady cadence of our footsteps, the rise and fall of our breath, the shifting landscapes that unfold before us - these sensations create a meditative state that can be truly restorative.

There is something about being out in the open air, surrounded by natural beauty, that has a profoundly calming and uplifting effect.

Whether it's a leisurely stroll through a park, a vigorous hike up a mountain trail, or a brisk walk to run errands, the act of putting one foot in front of the other can unlock a profound sense of joy and freedom. With each step, we shed the stress and worries of daily life and reconnect with the simple pleasure of movement.

The specific joys of walking will vary from person to person. For some, it may be the thrill of exploring new environments and discovering hidden gems. For others, it could be the satisfaction of setting and achieving fitness goals. And for many, it is simply the blissful solitude of being alone with one's thoughts, surrounded by the beauty of the natural world.

Regardless of the individual motivations, there is no doubt that walking has the power to transform our lives in profound and nourishing ways. The next time you need a pick-me-up or a moment of respite, lace up your shoes, step outside, and let the joy of walking carry you away.

The Long-Term Impact of Walking:

Incorporating walking into your lifestyle has the potential to create a ripple effect of positive changes. As you experience the immediate joys and benefits of walking, you may find yourself inspired to adopt other healthy habits, such as eating a balanced diet or prioritizing self-care. Walking can serve as a gateway to a more active and fulfilling life, empowering you to take control of your health and well-being.

Moreover, the long-term impact of walking extends beyond the individual. Walking promotes a cleaner and greener environment, benefiting not only yourself but also future generations.

Walking is a simple yet powerful activity that holds the key to a healthier, happier, and more fulfilling life. By embracing the joy of walking, you embark on an amazing new adventure each day.

Chapter Two
10,000 Steps to a Greater Life

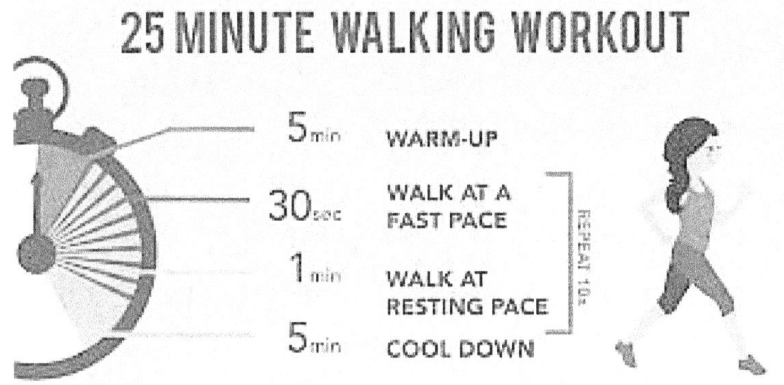

In today's sedentary world, where most people spend their days sitting at desks or lounging on couches, it is more important than ever to prioritize physical activity! One simple and effective way to increase your daily movement is by aiming to take between 400 and 10,000 steps a day. This small goal can have a profound impact on your overall health and well-being.

In this chapter we will explore the many advantages of taking between 400 and 10,000 steps a day and how it can transform your life. We will explore the many health benefits of making a commitment to take these extra steps every day. We will show you how to step your way to the best possible life ever!

10,000 steps a day – A simple step towards a healthier you!

In our fast-paced world, carving out time for exercise can feel like a luxury.

However, what if there was a way to significantly improve your health without needing a gym membership or having to spend hours with a sweaty workout?

Enter the power of walking! Aiming for 10,000 steps a day may seem daunting at first, but the benefits you will receive for your mental and physical wellbeing are undeniable.

It has been proven that with every 500 to 1000 extra steps you take is associated with a 15% reduction in the risk of dying from any cause!

An increase of just 500 steps a day was associated with a 7% reduction for dying from a cardiovascular disease, according to research done at the John Hopkins School of Medicine.

Researchers led by Maciej Banach, a professor of cardiology at the Medical University of Lodz, Poland found that people that walked as many as 20,000 steps a day continued to have increased benefits, meaning that there is no upper limit. The more steps you take in a day, the more benefits you will realize!

"Our study confirms that the more you walk, the better", says Prof. Banach. "We found that this applies to both men and women, irrespective of age, and irrespective of whether you live in a temperate, sub-tropical or sub-polar region of the world, or a region with a mixture of climates. In addition, our analysis indicates that as little as 4,000 steps a day are needed to significantly reduce deaths from any cause, and even fewer steps can reduce deaths from cardiovascular disease.

In older adults, there was a 42% reduction in risk seen in those who walked between 6,000 and 10,000 steps a day, while there was a 49% reduction in risk in younger adults who walked between 7,000 and 13,000 steps a day.

The impact of step counts was not tested on people with different diseases, as the participants were generally healthy when they entered the studies analyzed.

Getting 9,000 to 10,000 steps a day lowered the risk of cardiovascular diseaste by 21%, and the odds dying early by 39% according to a study published by the British Journal of Sports Medicine.

According to World Health Organization data, insufficient physical activity is the fourth most frequent cause of death in the world, with 3.2 MILLION deaths a year related to physical inactivity.

Walking is a favorite form of exercise for many people, and it's easy to see why. You can seamlessly fit it into your daily routine, walk to the beat of your favorite tunes, or do it while catching up with a good friend (or even a group). Just think about it—you don't need a gym membership to start walking and there are some great routes just waiting to be explored right outside your front door.

Studies suggest that walking can significantly reduce the risk of developing chronic diseases like type 2 diabetes and certain types of cancer.

Walking is also a weight-bearing exercise, meaning it forces your muscles and bones to work against gravity. This helps build stronger bones and improves joint health, reducing the risk of osteoporosis and arthritis.

Getting steps in each day is an excellent way to burn calories. As a matter of fact, engaging in regular physical activity like going on walks is key to maintaining a healthy weight. "Walking is beneficial because it adds to the overall daily calorie expenditure, which will eventually add to weight loss," explains April Gatlin, master coach for Stride Fitness. "Walking is also beneficial because it can be done by anyone with minimal equipment!"

If you're a newbie to the walking game, don't fret. Feel free to kickstart your journey with some short walks at a light intensity. You can gradually increase the lengths and intensity of your walks as you progress.

As you're working your way toward your weight-loss goal, keep in mind that consistency is key. This includes all aspects of your regimen, from diet to exercise. "Consistency is the only way you will see progress towards the weight loss goal," So do whatever you need to do to carve out some time during your day to head out on an invigorating walk—no excuses!

Wearable tech

Using the latest technology is an excellent way to track your progress, motivate yourself, and hold yourself accountable. Whether you invest in a Fitbit, Apple Watch, or Garmin, or use a walking app/fitness tracker on your phone, this is a smart addition to your daily fitness regimen.

Get a little bit "uncomfortable." This doesn't mean pushing yourself to the max when you're just starting out, but rather, when you feel you're ready, pick up the pace! "Your pace should be quick (not just a leisurely stroll-in-the-park) where the heart rate is elevated.

Mike Bohl, MD, and a certified personal trainer and nutrition coach, suggests varying the terrain you walk on. Doing your walks on a flat, paved surface is all well and good. But to give your body more of a challenge and promote weight loss, consider switching up the terrain.

'Anywhere you can go that has rolling hills (or even steep hills) can increase your calorie burn, and walking on some surfaces, like sand, can also take extra effort and burn more calories.'

Tyler Read, the founder of PTPioneer.com and a personal trainer who has been involved in health and fitness for the past 15 years, agrees that opting for a trail over flat pavement is a solid course of action. "Trails require more stabilizing of muscles and they are more energy demanding," he explains.

Do Interval Walking

The varied paces in interval walking enhance your body's ability to deliver oxygen to muscles. "Adding higher-intensity intervals pushes your cardiovascular system to work harder, which means it will adapt to the new challenge by becoming more efficient," says Rachel MacPherson, CPT, an ACE-certified personal trainer. with Garage Gym "This is how you get fitter, and you can push harder next time. It's also how you improve your cardiovascular health, which means lower risks of heart disease, stroke and dementia," she says.

Chapter Three
Walking for Extreme Creativity

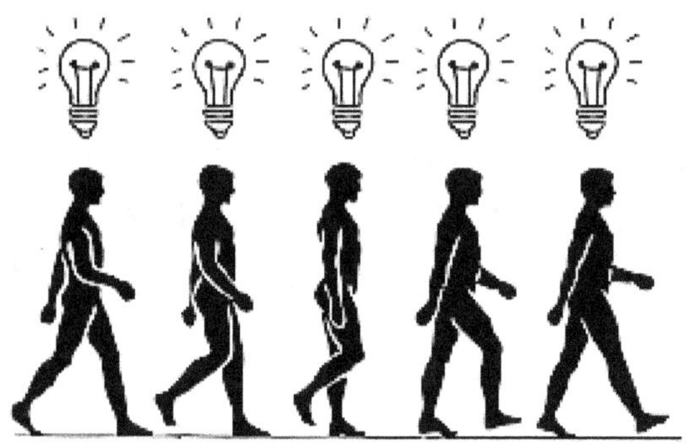

Walking is "a state in which the mind, the body, and the world are aligned," and Thomas Bernhard's insight that "there is nothing more revealing than to see a thinking person walking, just as there is nothing more revealing than to see a walking person thinking," and Wind in the Willows author Kenneth Grahame's insistence that solitary walks "set the mind jogging… make it garrulous, exalted, a little mad maybe — certainly creative and supersensitive," and of course it was Thoreau, who believed that "every walk is a sort of crusade" for returning to our senses.

So why is walking so conducive to creativity?

There are several reasons:

Increased blood flow to the brain: Walking gets your blood pumping, which increases the flow of oxygen and nutrients to the brain. This enhanced blood flow has been linked to improved cognitive function, including creative thinking.

Reduced stress and anxiety: Walking, especially in natural environments, has a calming effect on the mind and body. It reduces levels of the stress hormone cortisol and promotes the release of endorphins, the body's natural mood-boosters. Lower stress levels allow the mind to relax and wander, which is essential for creative insights to emerge.

Stimulation of the default mode network: Walking activates the brain's default mode network, a set of interconnected brain regions that are active when we are not focused on external tasks. This network is associated with daydreaming, imagination, and self-reflection - all key components of the creative process.

Exposure to new stimuli: When we walk, especially outdoors, we encounter a constantly changing environment full of new sights, sounds, and sensations. This exposure to novel stimuli can spark new ideas and associations in the brain, fueling creative thinking.

Rhythmic motion: The steady, rhythmic motion of walking may help to synchronize the left and right hemispheres of the brain, leading to improved communication and collaboration between the logical and creative sides of the brain.

How to Walk Your Way to Extreme Creativity

Now that we understand the science behind walking and creativity, let's explore some practical ways to incorporate more walking into your daily routine for maximum creative benefits:

Take a daily creativity walk: Set aside dedicated time each day for a "creativity walk." This could be a 20–30-minute walk in the morning, during your lunch break, or in the evening. Use this time to let your mind wander and explore new ideas without any specific agenda.

Walk during brainstorming sessions: Instead of sitting around a conference table, take your team on a walking brainstorming session. Walking side by side can break down hierarchical barriers and promote a more open, collaborative atmosphere. Plus, the change of scenery and physical movement can help generate fresh perspectives and ideas.

Use walking to overcome creative blocks: When you feel stuck on a problem or project, go for a walk. The physical act of walking can help shift your mental state and allow new insights to emerge. Often, the solution will come to you when you least expect it, during or after your walk.

Vary your walking routes and environments: To maximize the creative benefits of walking, seek out diverse environments and routes. Walk in nature, explore new neighborhoods, or visit art galleries and museums. Exposing yourself to new stimuli and experiences can broaden your perspective and inspire new ideas.

Walk with a notebook or voice recorder: Capture your creative insights and ideas as they arise during your walks. Carry a small notebook and pen or use a voice recording app on your phone to quickly jot down or dictate your thoughts before they fade away.

Integrate walking into your work routine: Look for opportunities to incorporate walking into your workday. Take walking meetings, use a standing or treadmill desk, or simply take short walking breaks every hour to refresh your mind and body.

The simple act of walking can have a profound impact on your creativity and ability to generate new ideas. Many of history's greatest thinkers, writers, and innovators were avid walkers who used their daily strolls to stimulate their minds and imaginations.

Walking and Creativity: Unleashing the Power of Movement

Walking has long been celebrated for its physical benefits, from improving cardiovascular health to boosting mood and reducing stress. However, its connection to creativity is a fascinating aspect that has gained attention in recent years. Many renowned thinkers and artists have extolled the virtues of walking as a catalyst for creativity, citing its ability to stimulate the mind, foster introspection, and inspire new ideas. In this article, we delve into the profound link between walking and creativity, exploring how a simple act of putting one foot in front of the other can unlock a world of imagination and innovation.

The Rhythm of Movement and Mental Flow

Walking is a rhythmic activity that engages both body and mind in a harmonious dance. The repetitive motion of walking creates a soothing rhythm that can quiet the chatter of everyday life and allow thoughts to flow freely. This rhythmic movement has a meditative quality, similar to the practice of mindfulness or deep breathing exercises, which can help calm the mind and enhance focus.

Research has shown that walking promotes the production of neurotransmitters like dopamine and endorphins, which are associated with feelings of pleasure and well-being. These neurochemicals not only elevate mood but also contribute to a state of mental openness and receptivity. As a result, walkers often experience a heightened sense of creativity and problem-solving ability while on the move.

Nature's Influence on Creativity

Walking outdoors, especially in natural settings like parks, forests, or along scenic trails, amplifies the creative benefits of walking. Nature has a profound impact on our cognitive functioning, with studies demonstrating that exposure to natural environments can enhance creativity, improve cognitive performance, and increase feelings of vitality.

The concept of "biophilia," proposed by biologist Edward O. Wilson, suggests that humans have an innate connection to nature and derive psychological benefits from interacting with natural elements. When we walk in natural surroundings, our senses are enlivened by the sights, sounds, and smells of the environment. This sensory stimulation not only invigorates the mind but also sparks imaginative thinking and creative insights.

The Mind-Wandering Effect

Walking is conducive to mind-wandering, a cognitive state characterized by spontaneous and unconstrained thoughts. Unlike focused attention tasks that require concentrated effort, mind-wandering allows the mind to wander freely, making unexpected connections and generating novel ideas.

Psychological studies have found that mind-wandering is closely linked to creativity, as it enables the brain to engage in associative thinking and divergent thought patterns. When walking, the gentle rhythm of movement combined with the tranquil surroundings encourages the mind to drift, leading to moments of insight and creative breakthroughs.

Walking as a Ritual of Inspiration

For many creative individuals, walking serves as a ritual of inspiration—a deliberate practice that primes the mind for creative work. Writers, artists, and innovators throughout history have embraced walking as part of their creative process, using it to incubate ideas, overcome creative blocks, and gain fresh perspectives.

Walking allows for uninterrupted solitude, providing a space for introspection and reflection. This solitude is essential for creativity, as it allows the mind to wander freely without external distractions. As thoughts meander during a walk, unrelated ideas converge, sparking new concepts and imaginative leaps.

Incorporating Walking into Your Creative Routine

If you're looking to harness the creative power of walking, consider integrating walking into your daily routine in the following ways:

Walking Meetings: Instead of traditional sit-down meetings, opt for walking meetings outdoors. The movement and change of scenery can stimulate creativity and enhance collaboration.

Mindful Walking: Practice mindful walking by focusing your attention on each step, the sensations in your body, and the surrounding environment. This mindful awareness can deepen your connection to creativity.

Walking Breaks: Take short walking breaks throughout the day to clear your mind, recharge your energy, and invite new ideas.

Creative Walks: Dedicate specific walks to creative exploration, whether brainstorming ideas, drafting narratives, or visualizing artistic concepts.

By incorporating walking into your creative routine, you can tap into a rich source of inspiration, enhance cognitive flexibility, and unleash your creative potential. Whether strolling through nature's splendor or pacing the city streets, each step can be a catalyst for creativity, leading to innovative breakthroughs and artistic expression.

Walking is not just a physical activity; it's a journey of the mind and spirit. Its profound effects on creativity stem from its ability to synchronize body and mind, engage with nature's beauty, foster mind-wandering, and serve as a ritual of inspiration. As you lace up your shoes and embark on a walk, remember that every step is a stride toward unlocking the boundless creativity that resides within you.

Chapter Four
Interval Walking

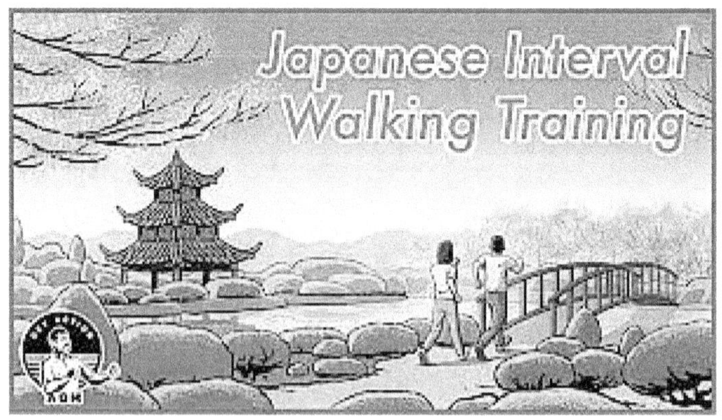

Interval walking is an exercise technique that alternates periods of high-intensity walking with lower-intensity walking or rest. This form of exercise is gaining popularity for its effectiveness in improving cardiovascular health, aiding in weight loss, and enhancing overall fitness levels. Whether you're a seasoned athlete or a beginner looking to improve your health, interval walking can be tailored to meet your specific needs and goals. This article will explore the benefits, techniques, and tips for incorporating interval walking into your fitness routine.

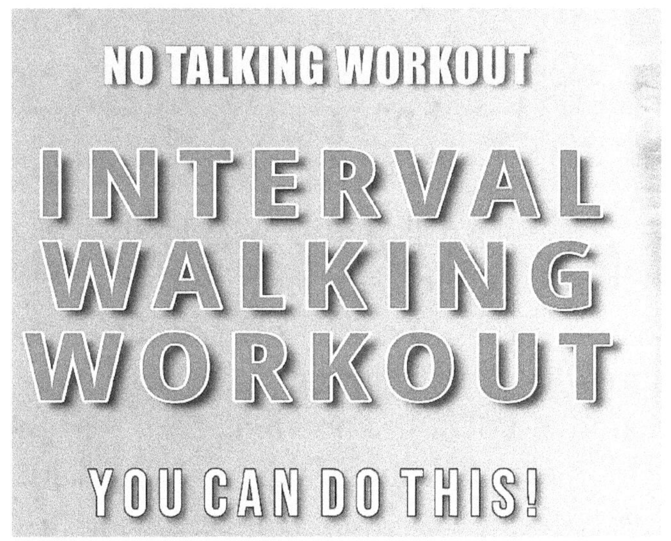

The Benefits of Interval Walking

Improved Cardiovascular Health

One of the primary benefits of interval walking is its positive impact on cardiovascular health. By alternating between high-intensity and low-intensity walking, you challenge your heart and lungs, leading to improved cardiovascular endurance. This type of exercise increases your heart rate during the high-intensity intervals, enhancing heart function and circulation. Over time, this can lead to a lower resting heart rate and reduced risk of cardiovascular diseases.

Enhanced Weight Loss

Interval walking is an effective strategy for weight loss. The bursts of high-intensity activity increase your metabolism, leading to greater calorie burn both during and after your workout. This phenomenon, known as the afterburn effect, means your body continues to burn calories at an elevated rate even after you've finished exercising. Additionally, the varying intensities can prevent workout monotony, making it easier to stay committed to your fitness goals.

Increased Muscle Tone and Strength

Incorporating high-intensity intervals into your walking routine engages more muscle groups than steady-state walking. The increased effort during these intervals helps to build and tone muscles in your legs, glutes, and core. Over time, this can lead to improved muscle strength and endurance, enhancing your overall physical fitness.

Improved Insulin Sensitivity

Interval walking can also have a positive impact on insulin sensitivity, which is crucial for managing blood sugar levels. Studies have shown that high-intensity interval training (HIIT) can improve the body's ability to use insulin effectively, reducing the risk of type 2 diabetes. By incorporating interval walking into your routine, you can help regulate blood sugar levels and improve metabolic health.

Techniques for Interval Walking
Choosing the Right Intervals

The key to effective interval walking is finding the right balance between high-intensity and low-intensity periods. Beginners might start with shorter high-intensity intervals, such as 30 seconds to 1 minute, followed by 1 to 2 minutes of low-intensity walking. As your fitness level improves, you can gradually increase the duration and intensity of your high-intensity intervals.

Warm-Up and Cool-Down

As with any exercise routine, it's essential to include a proper warm-up and cool-down. Start with 5-10 minutes of light walking to prepare your muscles and cardiovascular system for the workout. After completing your intervals, spend another 5-10 minutes walking at a slower pace to help your body gradually return to its resting state. This can prevent injuries and reduce post-workout soreness.

Varying Terrain and Speed

To keep your workouts interesting and challenging, vary the terrain and speed of your intervals. Incorporate hills, stairs, or different walking surfaces to engage different muscle groups and add intensity. You can also experiment with different walking speeds, from brisk walking to power walking, to keep your body guessing and prevent plateaus.

Monitoring Intensity

It's important to monitor your intensity during interval walking to ensure you're getting the most out of your workout. You can use a heart rate monitor or the talk test to gauge your exertion level. During high-intensity intervals, you should be working hard enough that talking becomes difficult, but you can still speak a few words. During low-intensity intervals, you should be able to carry on a conversation more comfortably.

Tips for Successful Interval Walking

Set Realistic Goals

Setting realistic and achievable goals is crucial for staying motivated and tracking your progress. Start with small, attainable goals, such as completing a certain number of intervals or increasing your walking speed. As you reach these goals, gradually set more challenging ones to keep pushing yourself.

Listen to Your Body

While interval walking is an excellent way to improve fitness, it's important to listen to your body and avoid overtraining. Pay attention to any signs of fatigue, pain, or discomfort, and adjust your intervals accordingly. It's better to progress slowly and steadily than to risk injury by pushing yourself too hard.

Stay Hydrated and Nourished

Proper hydration and nutrition are essential for optimal performance and recovery. Make sure to drink plenty of water before, during, and after your workouts to stay hydrated. Eating a balanced diet rich in proteins, carbohydrates, and healthy fats will provide the necessary fuel for your body to perform and recover effectively.

Use Proper Footwear

Wearing the right shoes can make a significant difference in your interval walking experience. Choose walking shoes that provide good support, cushioning, and traction. This will help prevent injuries and make your workouts more comfortable and enjoyable.

Incorporating Interval Walking into Your Routine

Start Slowly

If you're new to interval walking, start slowly and gradually increase the intensity and duration of your intervals. Begin with a simple routine, such as 30 seconds of brisk walking followed by 1-2 minutes of slow walking. As you become more comfortable, you can increase the intensity and length of the high-intensity intervals.

Mix It Up

To prevent boredom and keep your workouts effective, mix up your interval walking routine. Change the duration and intensity of your intervals, try new routes, and incorporate different types of terrain. This variety will keep you motivated and help you achieve better results.

Track Your Progress

Keeping track of your progress can be incredibly motivating. Use a fitness tracker or a journal to record your workouts, including the duration, intensity, and distance covered. Seeing your improvements over time can boost your confidence and encourage you to keep goin

Interval walking is a versatile and effective form of exercise that offers numerous health benefits, from improved cardiovascular health and weight loss to increased muscle tone and insulin sensitivity. By incorporating intervals of high intensity walking into your routine, you can challenge your body in new ways and achieve better fitness results. Whether you're a beginner or an experienced walker, interval walking can be adapted to suit your fitness level and goals. So, lace up your walking shoes, set your intervals, and start reaping the rewards of this dynamic exercise technique.

Chapter Five
Walking as a Way of Life

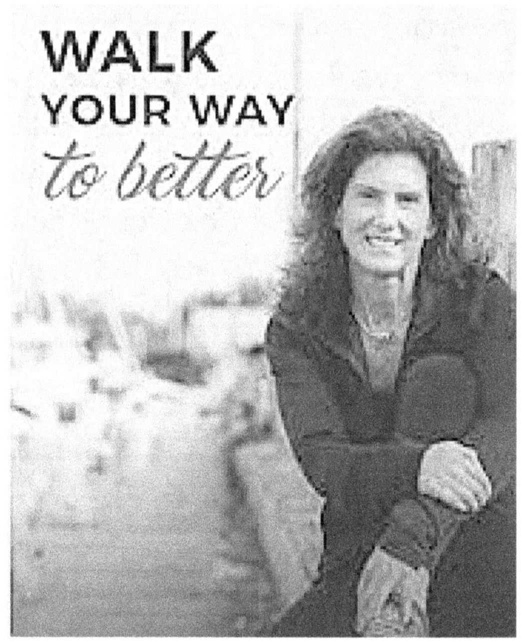

For many of us, walking is simply a means of getting from point A to point B. But what if walking became more than just a mode of transportation? What if it became a central part of how you live your life each day?

In this chapter, we'll explore the profound benefits that come from making walking a daily habit and an integral part of your lifestyle. Beyond just the physical health advantages, walking can transform your mental well-being, creativity, relationships, and connection to the world around you.

We'll look at ways to seamlessly work more walking into your existing routines and responsibilities. From walking meetings at work to evening walks with family to multi-day walking adventures, you'll get practical tips on how to step up your walking game.

The goal is to make walking feel less like an "exercise chore" and more like a natural, energizing and life-enriching part of your day. Discover the joy and rewards that come from slowing down, lacing up your shoes, and experiencing life one step at a time. By the end of this chapter, you will be inspired to embrace walking not just as an activity, but as a critical part of your life.

One of the simplest and most effective ways to improve your overall health and well-being is often overlooked: that is walking. Walking is a low-impact, accessible form of exercise that can be easily incorporated into your daily routine. Not only does it provide numerous physical health benefits, but it also contributes to better mental health and can even lead to a longer life. In the following pages, we will explore the various ways in which walking can improve your health. We will also provide practical tips on how to make walking a regular part of your life.

Walking burns calories and can help you maintain a healthy weight. By incorporating walking into your daily routine, you can prevent weight gain and support weight loss efforts when combined with a balanced diet. Even a moderate pace of walking can burn a significant number of calories over time.

Muscle Strength and Joint Health:

Walking engages multiple muscle groups in your legs, core, and upper body. It helps strengthen and tone these muscles, improving overall strength and stability. Additionally, walking is a low-impact exercise that is gentle on your joints, making it suitable for people of all ages and fitness levels. It can help alleviate joint pain and stiffness associated with conditions like arthritis.

Bone Density

Weight-bearing exercises, such as walking, can help maintain and improve bone density. This is particularly important for older adults, as bone density naturally decreases with age, increasing the risk of osteoporosis and fractures. Regular walking can help slow down bone loss and reduce the risk of age-related bone conditions.

Immune System Boost

Walking has been shown to enhance immune function. It increases the circulation of immune cells throughout the body, helping to fight off infections and diseases more effectively. Regular walking can also reduce inflammation in the body, which is linked to various chronic health conditions.

Mental Health Benefits

Walking has a calming effect on the mind and can help reduce stress and anxiety. It provides an opportunity to step away from daily stressors, clear your thoughts, and enjoy some quiet time. The rhythmic motion of walking and being in nature can promote relaxation and lower cortisol levels, the stress hormone.

Mood Enhancement

Exercise, including walking, releases endorphins, the body's natural mood-boosting chemicals. Regular walking can help alleviate symptoms of depression and improve overall mood. It can also increase self-esteem and confidence, as you set and achieve walking goals.

Cognitive Function

Walking has been linked to improved cognitive function and brain health. It increases blood flow to the brain, providing it with oxygen and nutrients. This can enhance memory, concentration, and overall brain function. Regular walking may also reduce the risk of age-related cognitive decline and dementia.

Creativity and Problem-Solving

Walking, especially in natural environments, can stimulate creativity and aid in problem-solving. The change of scenery and the repetitive motion of walking can help generate new ideas and perspectives. Many people find that going for a walk helps them think more clearly and come up with solutions to challenges they face.

Longevity and Quality of Life

Studies have shown that regular walking is associated with increased longevity and a better quality of life. People who walk regularly tend to live longer and have a lower risk of chronic diseases compared to those who are sedentary. Walking can help maintain independence and mobility as you age, allowing you to engage in daily activities with ease.

Chapter Six
Walking Will Transform Your Life

Walking, a simple yet profound activity, offers more than just a means to get from one place to another. It has the power to inspire, to heal, and to transform. Whether it's a leisurely stroll through a park, a brisk walk-through city streets, or a hike through nature, walking can open up new perspectives, stimulate creativity, and provide a sense of peace and clarity.

Walking is one of the simplest yet most powerful activities you can do to improve your physical health, mental wellbeing, and overall quality of life. The simple act of putting one foot in front of the other and moving your body through space can have profound transformative effects. Here are some of the key ways that walking will change you for the better:

Walking is not only beneficial for the mind but also for the body. It is a form of exercise that can improve physical health, boost mood, and reduce stress. The physical act of walking releases endorphins, which are natural mood enhancers. This chemical reaction in the brain can help to alleviate anxiety and depression, leading to a more positive outlook on life.

Moreover, walking in natural environments, such as parks or forests, can amplify these benefits. Nature walks have been shown to reduce cortisol levels, a hormone associated with stress, and increase feelings of well-being. The sights, sounds, and smells of nature can be incredibly soothing, providing a sensory experience that can ground us in the present moment and inspire a sense of awe and wonder.

The Historical and Cultural Significance of Walking

Throughout history, walking has been a fundamental part of human existence. Ancient philosophers like Socrates and Aristotle walked as they taught, believing that movement stimulated thought. The tradition of walking as a means of intellectual and spiritual exploration continued with figures like Henry David Thoreau, who wrote extensively about his walks in nature. Thoreau's walks were not just physical journeys but also journeys of the mind, where he found inspiration in the natural world around him.

In many cultures, walking is also seen as a pilgrimage, a journey with a sacred or significant purpose. The Camino de Santiago in Spain, for instance, is a famous pilgrimage route that attracts thousands of walkers each year, seeking spiritual growth, personal reflection, and a sense of accomplishment. These historical and cultural contexts highlight walking's deep connection to inspiration and personal growth.

Improved Physical Health

Regular walking strengthens your heart, lungs, bones, and muscles. It lowers blood pressure, improves circulation, and reduces the risk of chronic diseases like obesity, diabetes, heart disease, and some cancers. Walking burns calories to help maintain a healthy weight. It also improves balance, coordination, and joint mobility, especially important as you age. Just 30 minutes of brisk walking most days delivers significant health benefits.

Boosted Mood and Mental Wellbeing

Walking, especially outdoors, is a natural mood booster. It reduces stress, anxiety, and symptoms of depression by releasing endorphins - your body's feel-good chemicals. A daily walk clears your head, lifts your spirits, and helps put problems in perspective. Walking in nature is especially beneficial for mental health. It increases focus and creativity while reducing rumination on negative thoughts. Walking while socializing with a friend combines the benefits of exercise, fresh air, and social connection.

Increased Energy and Productivity

Although it may seem counterintuitive, expending energy on a walk increases your overall energy levels throughout the day. Walking boosts circulation and oxygen supply to all your tissues, helping you feel more alert and energized. It also improves sleep quality, so you feel more rested. The mental clarity and focus that come from walking enable you to be more productive and efficient in your daily tasks. You'll get more done and feel better doing it.

Expanded Horizons and Perspectives

Walking takes you to new places, literally and figuratively. It enables you to explore your surroundings, see new sights, and break out of your usual routine. This opens up fresh perspectives and sparks new ideas. Walking also facilitates social interactions, whether it's greeting neighbors, making a new friend, or learning something interesting by walking with a companion. These connections and changes in outlook broaden your world and enrich your life experience.

As you can see, walking is a transformative activity that improves your life across multiple dimensions - physical, mental, social, and more. It is a simple pleasure with far-reaching effects. By making walking a regular habit, you'll be taking important strides toward a healthier body, happier mind, and better quality of life overall. The benefits will start from your very first step and only increase over your lifetime walking journey. So, lace up your shoes, step outside, and begin your positive transformation today.

Walking is often overlooked as a simple activity, something we do every day without much thought. Yet, beneath its apparent simplicity lies a transformative power that can profoundly impact our physical, mental, and emotional well-being. In this article, we delve into the myriad ways in which walking can truly transform your life.

The Power of Movement

At its core, walking is a fundamental form of human movement. From the moment we learn to take our first steps, walking becomes an integral part of our daily existence. Unlike more strenuous exercises, walking is accessible to everyone, regardless of age, fitness level, or physical condition. It doesn't require special equipment or training, making it one of the most inclusive forms of physical activity.

Physical Transformation

The benefits of walking for physical health are well-documented. Regular walking can improve cardiovascular fitness, strengthen muscles, and enhance flexibility. It is a low-impact exercise that puts less stress on joints compared to activities like running or weightlifting, making it ideal for those with joint pain or arthritis.

Moreover, walking outdoors exposes you to natural sunlight, boosting vitamin D levels and contributing to overall bone health.

Mental Clarity and Creativity

Beyond its physical benefits, walking has a profound impact on mental well-being. Many people find that walking helps clear their mind and reduce stress. The rhythmic movement of walking, combined with exposure to nature, can have a calming effect on the brain, leading to improved mood and mental clarity. Research also suggests that walking enhances creativity, with many writers, artists, and thinkers citing walks as a source of inspiration for their work.

Emotional Resilience

Walking can also foster emotional resilience and psychological well-being. Engaging in regular walking routines can reduce symptoms of anxiety and depression, providing a natural mood boost. The sense of accomplishment from completing a walk, even a short one, can boost self-esteem and confidence. Additionally, walking in green spaces or natural environments has been linked to greater feelings of happiness and connectedness to the world around us.

Social Connection

Walking has a unique ability to foster social connections and build communities. Walking clubs, group hikes, or simply walking with friends or family members can strengthen relationships and create shared experiences. The act of walking side by side encourages conversations and bonding, leading to a sense of belonging and support. In an increasingly digital world, where virtual connections often dominate, walking offers a tangible way to connect with others in real life.

Lifestyle Integration

One of the most significant advantages of walking is its ease of integration into daily life. Unlike gym workouts that require dedicated time and effort, walking can be incorporated into your existing routine. Whether it's walking to work, taking a stroll during lunch breaks, or exploring nature trails on weekends, there are countless opportunities to add more steps to your day. This seamless integration makes walking a sustainable and enjoyable long-term habit.

Environmental Impact

Aside from personal benefits, walking also has a positive impact on the environment. Choosing to walk instead of driving reduces carbon emissions and helps preserve natural resources. By embracing walking as a primary mode of transportation whenever possible, individuals can contribute to a greener, more sustainable planet.

Walking is not just a mundane activity but a powerful catalyst for transformation. It has the potential to improve physical health, enhance mental clarity and creativity, foster emotional resilience, build social connections, integrate seamlessly into daily life, and contribute to a healthier planet. Whether you're taking leisurely strolls in the park or embarking on challenging hikes, every step you take brings you closer to a transformed life. So, lace up your shoes, step outside, and let walking guide you on a journey of personal growth and well-being.

The Mind-Body Connection

Mindfulness is the practice of being fully present and engaged in the current moment, and walking can be an excellent way to cultivate this state of awareness. Mindful walking involves paying attention to the sensations of each step, the movement of the body, and the environment around us. This practice can help to quiet the mind, reduce distractions, and increase focus.

When we walk mindfully, we become more attuned to our surroundings and our inner experiences. This heightened awareness can lead to a deeper appreciation of the beauty and intricacy of the world around us. It can also help us to connect with our inner selves, fostering a sense of clarity and insight. By incorporating mindfulness into our walking routine, we can transform a simple walk into a meditative and inspiring experience.

Finding Inspiration in Everyday Walks

You don't need to embark on a grand adventure or travel to a far-off destination to find inspiration in walking. Everyday walks, whether they are in your neighborhood, a local park, or even a city street, can be equally inspiring. The key is to approach these walks with an open and curious mind, ready to observe and appreciate the details of your surroundings.

Consider taking different routes, exploring new areas, or walking at different times of the day to experience your environment in various ways. Notice the changing seasons, the architecture, the people you pass by, and the small moments of beauty that often go unnoticed. These everyday walks can provide a fresh perspective, spark new ideas, and remind us of the richness of our daily lives.

Walking for Personal Growth

Walking can also inspire personal growth and self-discovery. It offers an opportunity for introspection and reflection, allowing us to gain insights into our thoughts, emotions, and experiences. The solitude and tranquility of a walk can create a space for self-examination and the exploration of our inner landscape.

As we walk, we can contemplate our goals, aspirations, and the challenges we face. This reflective process can help us to gain clarity, find solutions, and develop a greater understanding of ourselves. Walking can also inspire us to set new intentions, make positive changes, and pursue our passions with renewed vigor.

The Community Aspect of Walking

While walking can be a solitary activity, it can also be a communal one. Walking with others can foster a sense of connection and shared experience. Group walks, whether they are organized hikes, walking clubs, or casual strolls with friends and family, can provide a sense of camaraderie and support.

The conversations that occur during these walks can be enriching and inspiring. Sharing thoughts, ideas, and experiences with others can broaden our perspectives and deepen our understanding of the world. Walking with others can also motivate us to stay active and committed to our walking routine, creating a positive feedback loop of inspiration and well-being.

Walking is a simple yet powerful activity that has the potential to inspire us in myriad ways. It can enhance creativity, improve mental and physical health, foster mindfulness, and provide opportunities for personal growth and connection with others. By incorporating walking into our daily lives and approaching it with an open and curious mind, we can tap into its transformative potential and find inspiration in every step. Whether we are walking through city streets, natural landscapes, or familiar neighborhoods, walking can enrich our lives and lead us on a path of discovery, insight, and inspiration.

Chapter Seven
Walking Meditations

Why a Walking Meditation

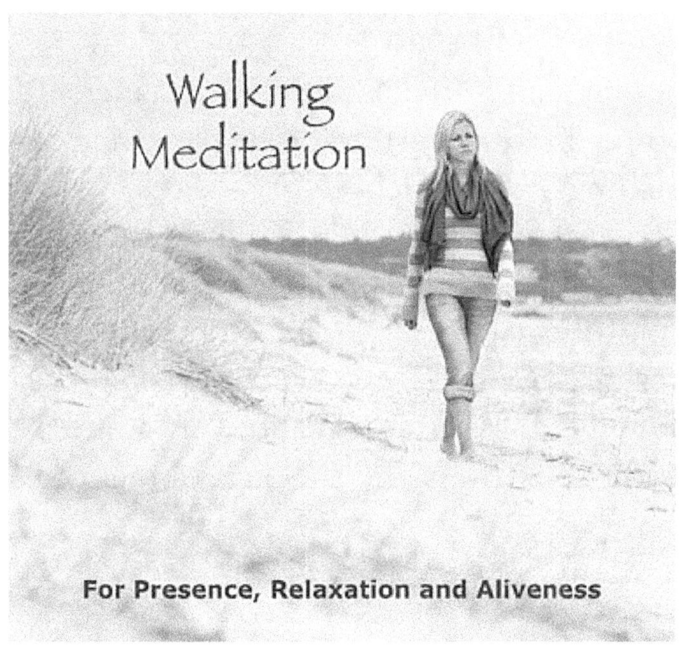

In a world where we are constantly bombarded with stimuli and stress, the search for tranquility and balance is more urgent than ever. While traditional seated meditation is well-known for its calming and centering effects, there is another form of meditation that combines mindfulness with physical movement: walking meditation. This practice offers a unique and powerful way to cultivate mindfulness, enhance physical health, and foster a deeper connection with oneself and the surrounding environment.

The Concept of Walking Meditation

Walking meditation is an ancient practice rooted in Buddhist traditions, particularly in the teachings of Thich Nhat Hanh, a renowned Vietnamese Zen master. Unlike seated meditation, walking meditation involves the deliberate and mindful act of walking. It emphasizes being fully present in each step, synchronizing breath with movement, and cultivating awareness of the body's sensations and the environment.

The Benefits of Walking Meditation

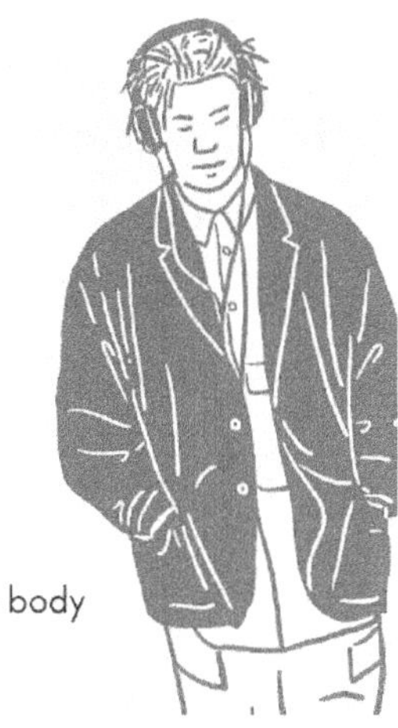

1. Mindfulness and Presence

Walking meditation invites practitioners to focus on the present moment, reducing the constant chatter of the mind. By paying attention to the sensation of each step, the rhythm of the breath, and the sounds and sights around, individuals can anchor themselves in the now. This mindfulness practice can help break the cycle of stress and anxiety, promoting a sense of calm and clarity.

2. Physical Health

The physical benefits of walking are well-documented. Regular walking can improve cardiovascular health, boost metabolism, and strengthen muscles and bones. Walking meditation combines these physical benefits with mental well-being. The gentle movement can also be particularly beneficial for those who find it challenging to sit still for extended periods, providing a way to engage in meditation without discomfort.

3. Emotional Regulation

Walking meditation can serve as a powerful tool for emotional regulation. The rhythmic movement and focus on the present can help individuals process emotions more effectively. It provides an opportunity to reflect and gain perspective, fostering emotional resilience and reducing feelings of overwhelm.

4. Enhanced Creativity and Problem-Solving

The combination of movement and mindfulness can stimulate creative thinking and problem-solving abilities. As the mind becomes more relaxed and open during walking meditation, new ideas and solutions can emerge. This practice can be particularly beneficial for those in creative fields or anyone seeking fresh perspectives on challenges.

5. Connection with Nature

Walking meditation often takes place outdoors, allowing practitioners to connect with nature. This connection can enhance the meditative experience, providing a sense of grounding and belonging. The natural world offers a soothing backdrop, helping to reduce stress and improve overall well-being.

How to Practice Walking Meditation

1. Find a Suitable Location

Choose a quiet, safe place where you can walk undisturbed. This could be a park, a garden, or even a quiet room. The path should be clear and free of obstacles to allow for mindful walking.

2. Set an Intention

Begin with an intention for your practice. This could be a specific focus, such as cultivating peace, letting go of stress, or simply being present. Setting an intention can help guide your practice and keep you focused.

3. Start Slowly

Start walking slowly and deliberately. Pay attention to the sensation of your feet touching the ground, the movement of your legs, and the rhythm of your breath. Keep your hands relaxed at your sides or gently clasped in front of you.

4. Synchronize Breath and Movement

Synchronize your breath with your steps. You might take a step with each inhale and another with each exhale, or take several steps with each breath. Find a rhythm that feels natural and calming for you.

5. Maintain Awareness

As you walk, maintain awareness of your surroundings. Notice the colors, sounds, and scents around you. If your mind wanders, gently bring your focus back to the sensation of walking and breathing.

6. Practice Regularly

Consistency is key in any meditation practice. Set aside regular time for walking meditation, whether it's a few minutes each day or longer sessions a few times a week. The more you practice, the deeper your experience will become.

Integrating Walking Meditation into Daily Life

Walking meditation is a versatile practice that can be integrated into daily life in various ways. Here are some tips on how to make walking meditation a regular part of your routine:

1. Morning Walks

Start your day with a mindful walk. This can set a positive tone for the day, helping you approach challenges with a calm and focused mind.

2. Breaks at Work

Take short walking meditation breaks during your workday. Step outside or find a quiet corridor to practice for a few minutes. This can help reduce stress and increase productivity.

3. Mindful Errands

Turn everyday errands into opportunities for walking meditation. Whether you're walking to the store or taking your dog for a walk, approach these activities with mindfulness.

4. Evening Strolls

End your day with a peaceful walk. This can help you unwind and reflect on the day, promoting better sleep and overall relaxation.

Walking meditation is a powerful practice that combines the benefits of physical activity with mindfulness. It offers a unique way to cultivate presence, enhance emotional and physical well-being, and connect with the world around us. By integrating walking meditation into our daily lives, we can find balance and peace in the midst of a busy world. Whether you are new to meditation or an experienced practitioner, walking meditation can provide a refreshing and enriching addition to your mindfulness practice.

Chapter Eight
Walking the Camino de Santiago Pilgrimage

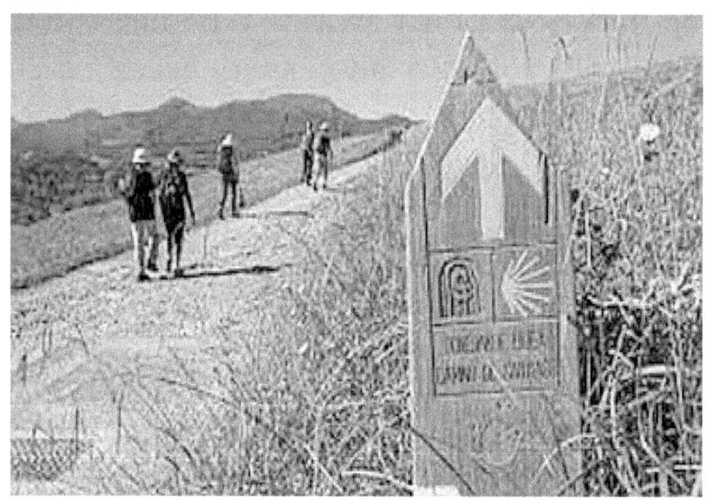

The Camino de Santiago, also known as the 'Way of St. James,' is a network of ancient pilgrimage routes leading to the shrine of the apostle Saint James the Great in the cathedral of Santiago de Compostela in Galicia, northwestern Spain. Every year, thousands of pilgrims and adventurers from all walks of life embark on this spiritual and physical journey, each with their own motivations and experiences. The Camino de Santiago is not just a walk; it is a transformative journey that combines history, culture, spirituality, and personal discovery.

A Historical Perspective

The origins of the Camino de Santiago date back to the 9th century when the remains of Saint James were discovered in Santiago de Compostela. The news of this miraculous find spread quickly, and Santiago became one of the most important Christian pilgrimage destinations, rivaling Rome and Jerusalem. Over the centuries, the pilgrimage route became well-trodden by devout Christians seeking penance, adventure, and a closer connection to their faith.

The Routes of the Camino

There are several routes to Santiago de Compostela, each offering unique landscapes, challenges, and experiences. The most popular route is the Camino Francés, which begins in St. Jean Pied de Port on the French side of the

Pyrenees and stretches approximately 780 kilometers to Santiago. This route takes pilgrims through diverse landscapes, from the rugged mountains of the Pyrenees to the flat plains of the Meseta and the lush, green hills of Galicia.

Other notable routes include the Camino Portugués, starting in Lisbon or Porto, which provides a scenic journey through Portugal's charming towns and cities before crossing into Spain. The Camino del Norte follows the northern coast of Spain, offering stunning views of the Bay of Biscay, while the Via de la Plata, starting in Seville, is a longer and less-traveled route that traverses the heart of Spain.

The Pilgrim Experience

Walking the Camino de Santiago is a deeply personal experience. Pilgrims, known as peregrinos, come from all over the world, each with their own reasons for undertaking the journey. For some, it is a spiritual quest, a way to connect with their faith or seek answers to life's big questions. For others, it is an adventure, a challenge to test their physical and mental endurance. Some walk in memory of a loved one, while others simply seek the camaraderie and sense of community that the Camino offers.

One of the unique aspects of the Camino is the sense of camaraderie among pilgrims. As they walk, they share their stories, support each other through difficult moments, and form bonds that often last long after the journey ends. The Camino is also marked by the kindness of locals, who provide food, shelter, and encouragement to weary travelers. This sense of community and shared purpose is one of the most cherished aspects of the pilgrimage.

The Physical and Mental Challenge

Walking the Camino de Santiago is no small feat. Pilgrims typically walk between 20 and 30 kilometers a day, carrying all their belongings on their backs. The journey can take anywhere from a few weeks to several months, depending on the route and the pace of the walker. The physical demands of the walk can be intense, with blisters, sore muscles, and fatigue being common companions. However, many pilgrims find that the mental challenges are even greater than the physical ones.

The solitude of walking for hours each day provides ample time for reflection and introspection. Many pilgrims report experiencing a range of emotions, from joy and gratitude to frustration and doubt. The repetitive nature of walking can be meditative, allowing pilgrims to clear their minds and connect with their inner selves. This mental journey is often as transformative as the physical one, leading to a greater sense of self-awareness and personal growth.

The Spiritual Journey

For many, the Camino de Santiago is a deeply spiritual journey. The path is dotted with churches, chapels, and shrines, providing pilgrims with numerous opportunities for prayer and reflection. The act of walking itself can become a form of moving meditation, allowing pilgrims to connect with the divine in a profound way. Many pilgrims describe moments of clarity and insight that come to them during the walk, as well as a deep sense of peace and fulfillment.

Reaching the cathedral in Santiago de Compostela is a moment of profound significance for many pilgrims. The final steps into the plaza, with the towering cathedral in view, are often accompanied by a flood of emotions—relief, joy, gratitude, and a sense of accomplishment. Many pilgrims attend the Pilgrim's Mass at the cathedral, where they can reflect on their journey and give thanks for the experiences and lessons they have gained along the way.

The Cultural Richness

The Camino de Santiago is also a journey through history and culture. Along the way, pilgrims pass through charming villages, historic towns, and vibrant cities, each with its own unique character and traditions. The route is lined with ancient monasteries, castles, and other historical sites that provide a glimpse into the rich history of the region. Pilgrims can sample local cuisine, from hearty stews and fresh seafood to the famous wines of Rioja and Galicia.

The Camino is also a melting pot of cultures, with pilgrims from all over the world walking together and sharing their traditions and experiences. This cultural exchange enriches the journey, providing pilgrims with a broader perspective and a deeper appreciation for the diversity of human experience.

Practical Considerations

Walking the Camino de Santiago requires careful planning and preparation. Pilgrims need to be physically fit and mentally prepared for the challenges of the journey. Choosing the right gear, including comfortable walking shoes and a well-fitted backpack, is essential. Pilgrims should also plan their route and accommodations in advance, as the popularity of the Camino means that hostels and albergues can fill up quickly, especially during peak season.

It's also important to be aware of the practical aspects of walking the Camino, such as staying hydrated, taking care of one's feet, and listening to one's body. Many pilgrims find that the journey is made easier by breaking it into manageable stages and allowing for rest days along the way.

The Camino de Santiago is more than just a walk; it is a journey of transformation. Whether undertaken for spiritual, personal, or recreational reasons, the Camino offers a unique opportunity to step out of one's daily life and embark on an adventure of self-discovery and growth. The physical, mental, and spiritual challenges of the journey are balanced by the beauty of the landscape, the richness of the culture, and the sense of community and camaraderie that define the Camino experience. For those who have walked its ancient paths, the Camino de Santiago remains a cherished and life-changing journey, a testament to the enduring power of pilgrimage.

Chapter Nine
Walking to Find Yourself

In the hustle and bustle of modern life, many people find themselves yearning for a deeper sense of purpose and connection. Amidst the cacophony of daily routines, it can be challenging to carve out moments for introspection and self-discovery. One powerful, yet often overlooked, method to embark on this journey of self-discovery is through walking. This simple, ancient practice has the potential to unlock profound insights and foster a deeper connection with oneself.

The Historical and Cultural Significance of Walking

Walking has long been a fundamental part of human existence. Our ancestors relied on walking as their primary mode of transportation, using it to migrate, explore, and survive. Over time, walking has evolved from a mere means of getting from one place to another into a rich cultural and spiritual practice. Pilgrimages, such as the Camino de Santiago in Spain or the Kumano Kodo in Japan, are prime examples of how walking can be a transformative experience, providing individuals with the time and space to reflect on their lives and connect with their inner selves.

The Science Behind Walking and Self-Discovery

Numerous studies have shown that walking has a profound impact on both physical and mental health. Physically, it improves cardiovascular health, boosts immune function, and enhances overall fitness. Mentally, walking has been proven to reduce stress, alleviate symptoms of depression and anxiety, and improve cognitive function. When we walk, our bodies release endorphins, which elevate our mood and create a sense of well-being. This physiological response can create the ideal conditions for introspection and self-reflection.

Moreover, walking stimulates creative thinking. A study conducted by Stanford University found that walking increases creative output by an average of 60%. This is because walking allows the mind to wander and engage in a state of "free-flow" thinking, which can lead to new insights and ideas. When we walk, especially in natural settings, our minds are free from the constant barrage of digital stimuli, allowing us to tap into our subconscious and explore our thoughts more deeply.

Mindful Walking: A Path to Inner Awareness

Mindful walking, a practice rooted in Buddhist traditions, involves walking with full awareness of each step and breath. This form of walking meditation encourages individuals to focus on the present moment, paying attention to the sensations of their body, the rhythm of their breath, and the environment around them. By cultivating mindfulness during walking, we can develop a heightened sense of self-awareness and clarity.

To practice mindful walking, find a quiet place where you can walk undisturbed. Begin by standing still, taking a few deep breaths, and grounding yourself in the present moment. As you start walking, pay attention to the sensations in your feet as they contact the ground. Notice the movement of your legs, the sway of your arms, and the rhythm of your breath. If your mind starts to wander, gently bring your focus back to the act of walking. This practice not only helps calm the mind but also allows for a deeper connection with oneself.

Walking in Nature: A Gateway to Self-Discovery

Nature has a unique way of facilitating self-discovery. Walking in natural settings, such as forests, mountains, or by the sea, can have a profound impact on our mental and emotional well-being. The Japanese practice of "shinrin-yoku" or "forest bathing" involves immersing oneself in the forest atmosphere, taking in the sights, sounds, and smells of nature. Research has shown that spending time in nature reduces cortisol levels, lowers blood pressure, and boosts mood.

When we walk in nature, we are reminded of the beauty and interconnectedness of the world around us. This sense of awe and wonder can inspire introspection and help us gain a new perspective on our lives. The natural world serves as a mirror, reflecting our inner thoughts and feelings. As we walk through the changing landscapes, we may find ourselves more attuned to our own inner landscapes, gaining insights into our desires, fears, and aspirations.

Walking Through Life's Challenges

Life is full of challenges, and walking can be a powerful tool for navigating them. When faced with difficult decisions, emotional turmoil, or periods of uncertainty, taking a walk can provide the clarity and perspective needed to move forward. The rhythmic act of walking can help process emotions, release tension, and clear the mind. As we walk, we often find that solutions to our problems become more apparent, and we gain a greater sense of resilience and strength.

Consider the example of famous walkers like Henry David Thoreau, who retreated to Walden Pond to live simply and immerse himself in nature. Thoreau's walks were not just physical journeys but also journeys of self-discovery and reflection. His writings, inspired by his walks, continue to resonate with readers seeking a deeper connection with themselves and the natural world.

Creating a Walking Practice for Self-Discovery

Incorporating walking into your daily routine can be a transformative practice for self-discovery. Here are some tips to help you get started:

> ➢ Set an Intention: Before you begin your walk, set a clear intention. It could be to gain clarity on a specific issue, to release stress, or simply to connect with yourself. Having a purpose can guide your walk and make it more meaningful.

> Choose Your Path: Select a walking route that resonates with you. It could be a local park, a nature trail, or even a quiet street in your neighborhood. The environment you choose can significantly impact your experience.

> Walk Without Distractions: Leave your phone and other distractions behind. Allow yourself to be fully present in the moment,

> Focusing on your surroundings and your inner thoughts.

> Listen to Your Body: Pay attention to how your body feels as you walk. Notice any areas of tension or discomfort and adjust your pace accordingly. Walking should be a pleasurable and nurturing experience.

> Reflect and Journal: After your walk, take some time to reflect on your experience. Journaling can be a

powerful tool for capturing your thoughts and insights. Write down any revelations or emotions that arose during your walk.

Walking is more than just a physical activity; it is a journey of self-discovery and transformation. By embracing the practice of walking, we can create the space and time needed to connect with our inner selves, gain clarity on our life's path, and cultivate a sense of peace and well-being. Whether through mindful walking, immersing ourselves in nature, or using walking as a tool to navigate life's challenges, we can unlock the profound potential of this simple yet powerful practice. So, put on your walking shoes, step outside, and embark on the journey to find yourself.

Chapter Ten
Walking: A Transformational Journey

Walking, a simple act that many take for granted, holds profound potential to transform lives. Whether it's a leisurely stroll through a park, a brisk walk in the morning, or a determined trek up a mountain trail, walking offers countless benefits that extend beyond physical fitness. It can be a journey of self-discovery, emotional healing, and spiritual growth.

Here we explore how walking serves as a transformational journey, enhancing various aspects of our lives.

Walking for Mental Health

The connection between physical activity and mental health is well-established. Walking offers unique mental health benefits:

Stress Reduction: Walking helps reduce stress by promoting the release of endorphins, the body's natural mood elevators. It provides an opportunity to clear the mind and escape daily pressures.

Anxiety and Depression: Regular walking has been shown to alleviate symptoms of anxiety and depression. It can serve as a natural antidepressant, helping to lift moods and improve overall emotional well-being.

Cognitive Function: Walking boosts cognitive function and creativity. It enhances memory, attention, and problem-solving skills. Studies have shown that walking can help delay the onset of dementia and Alzheimer's disease.

Emotional and Spiritual Growth

Walking can also be a powerful tool for emotional and spiritual growth. It offers a unique way to connect with oneself and the world:

Mindfulness and Meditation: Walking can be a form of moving meditation. Mindful walking encourages present-moment awareness, helping individuals to stay grounded and centered. It can be a time for reflection and introspection.

Emotional Healing: Walking through nature can be particularly therapeutic. The sights, sounds, and smells of the natural environment can soothe the soul and promote emotional healing. Nature walks can help individuals process grief, loss, and other emotional challenges.

Spiritual Connection: For many, walking is a spiritual practice. It can be a time to connect with a higher power, reflect on life's purpose, and find inner peace. Pilgrimages, such as the Camino de Santiago, highlight walking's potential for spiritual transformation.

Walking as a Social Activity

Walking can also enhance social connections and build community:

Social Bonding: Walking with friends, family, or community groups can strengthen social bonds. It provides an opportunity for meaningful conversations and shared experiences.

Community Engagement: Walking events and group walks can foster a sense of community. They bring people together, promote social interaction, and encourage a sense of belonging.

The Transformative Power of Walking Through Life's Challenges

Walking can be a powerful coping mechanism during life's challenges. Whether dealing with personal loss, career transitions, or health issues, walking can provide clarity and perspective:

Processing Change: Walking allows individuals to process changes and transitions. It offers a quiet space to think, reflect, and come to terms with new realities.

Problem-Solving: The rhythmic nature of walking can enhance creative thinking and problem-solving. It provides a break from routine, allowing for fresh perspectives and innovative solutions.

Resilience Building: Regular walking can build resilience by promoting physical and mental stamina. It teaches perseverance and the value of taking one step at a time.

Practical Tips for Making Walking a Transformational Journey

To harness the full potential of walking as a transformational journey, consider the following tips:

Set Intentions: Before you start walking, set an intention. Whether it's to clear your mind, solve a problem, or simply enjoy nature, having a purpose can make your walk more meaningful.

Practice Mindfulness: Pay attention to your surroundings, your breath, and your body's movements. Mindful walking can enhance the meditative and emotional benefits of your walk.

Explore New Paths: Change your walking routes to keep the experience fresh and exciting.

Exploring new places can stimulate creativity and provide new perspectives.

Walk Regularly: Consistency is key. Aim to walk regularly, whether daily or several times a week. The cumulative benefits of regular walking are substantial.

Join a Group: Consider joining a walking group or participating in community walks. The social aspect can enhance motivation and provide additional emotional benefits.

Embrace Nature: Whenever possible, walk in natural settings. The connection with nature can amplify the emotional and spiritual benefits of walking.

Walking is more than just a physical activity; it's a transformational journey that can enhance every aspect of our lives. From physical health to mental well-being, emotional healing, spiritual growth, and social connection, walking offers a holistic approach to personal transformation. By embracing walking as a regular practice, we can unlock its full potential and embark on a journey of self-discovery and growth. So, lace up your walking shoes, step outside, and let the transformational journey begin.

Chapter Eleven
Walking to Lose Weight
(Walk it Off!)

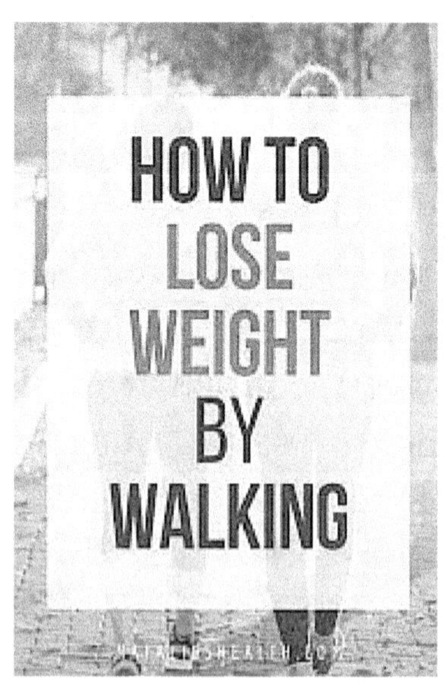

One of the most powerful benefits of walking is its ability to help you lose weight and maintain a healthy body composition. Walking is an accessible, low-impact form of exercise that can burn a significant number of calories when done regularly. By incorporating walking into your daily routine, you can boost your metabolism, reduce body fat, and achieve sustainable weight loss.

The number of calories burned while walking depends on several factors, including your weight, walking speed, and duration. On average, walking at a moderate pace of 3 miles per hour burns around 200-300 calories per hour for a 150-pound person. Increasing the intensity by walking faster, tackling hills or stairs, or using weights can further amplify the calorie-burning potential.

To lose one pound of body fat, you need to create a calorie deficit of approximately 3,500 calories. By walking for an hour each day, you can burn an extra 1,400 to 2,100 calories per week. Combined with a balanced diet, this can lead to a healthy weight loss of 1-2 pounds per week, which is a sustainable and recommended rate of weight loss.

In addition to burning calories, walking also helps to preserve lean muscle mass during weight loss. This is important because muscle tissue burns more calories at rest compared to fat tissue. By maintaining muscle through regular walking, you can keep your metabolism humming and make it easier to maintain your weight loss long-term.

Walking also helps to reduce stress, improve sleep quality, and boost overall mood and well-being - all of which can support healthy weight management. Chronic stress is linked to weight gain and emotional eating, so the stress-busting effects of walking can help you stay on track with your weight loss goals.

To maximize the weight loss benefits of walking, aim for at least 30 minutes of brisk walking most days of the week. You can break this up into shorter 10–15-minute sessions throughout the day if needed. Gradually increase your walking duration, frequency, and intensity over time to continue challenging your body and seeing results.

Remember, walking alone may not be enough for significant weight loss if your diet is not also balanced and calorie controlled. Combine regular walking with healthy eating habits for the best results. With consistency and dedication, walking can be a powerful tool in your weight loss journey, helping you shed pounds, boost your health, and feel your best.

Chapter Twelve
Walking for Strength and Flexibility

Walking, often perceived as a simple and leisurely activity, holds profound benefits for both physical and mental well-being. Beyond its cardiovascular advantages, walking plays a crucial role in enhancing strength and flexibility, making it a versatile exercise accessible to people of all ages and fitness levels. In this article, we delve into the science behind walking for strength and flexibility, exploring its impact on muscles, joints, and overall health.

The Basics of Walking as Exercise

At its core, walking is a weight-bearing exercise that involves the use of multiple muscles, joints, and bones. Unlike non-weight-bearing exercises like swimming or cycling, which are excellent for cardiovascular health but may not directly enhance bone density, walking provides a unique blend of cardiovascular stimulation and skeletal strengthening.

When you walk, especially at a brisk pace, your muscles contract and relax rhythmically, supporting the movement of your body. This repetitive action helps build endurance in your leg muscles, including the quadriceps, hamstrings, calves, and glutes. Over time, consistent walking can lead to improved muscle tone and strength in these areas.

Strengthening Muscles through Walking

One of the key benefits of walking for strength is its impact on the lower body muscles. Let's break down how walking strengthens specific muscle groups:

Quadriceps: These are the muscles at the front of your thighs. When you walk, especially uphill or at a faster pace, your quadriceps work harder to propel you forward and support your body weight.

Hamstrings: The muscles at the back of your thighs, the hamstrings, act as stabilizers during walking. They help control your leg movement and provide stability, especially when walking on uneven terrain.

Calves: Walking engages the calf muscles, particularly the gastrocnemius and soleus muscles. These muscles work to push off the ground with each step, contributing to the propulsion phase of walking.

Glutes: Your gluteal muscles, including the gluteus maximus, medius, and minimus, play a crucial role in walking. They help stabilize your pelvis, support your body's weight, and generate power during movements like climbing stairs or walking uphill.

By regularly engaging these muscle groups through walking, you can gradually increase their strength and endurance. This is especially beneficial for individuals looking to improve their lower body strength without high-impact exercises that can strain joints or lead to injuries.

Enhancing Flexibility through Walking

In addition to strength, walking also promotes flexibility in various ways:

Joint Mobility: Walking involves the movement of multiple joints, including the ankles, knees, hips, and spine. As you walk, these joints go through a range of motion, promoting joint flexibility and mobility. This is particularly beneficial for individuals with sedentary lifestyles or those recovering from injuries, as it helps prevent stiffness and maintains joint health.

Muscle Stretching: Walking, especially when combined with dynamic stretching exercises, can help stretch and lengthen muscles. As you stride and swing your arms while walking, your muscles undergo a gentle stretching action. This improves overall flexibility and reduces the risk of muscle tightness or cramps.

Postural Alignment: Proper posture is essential for flexibility and overall well-being. Walking with good posture, where your spine is aligned, shoulders are relaxed, and core muscles are engaged, contributes to better flexibility by optimizing the alignment of your musculoskeletal system.

Moreover, walking on varied terrain, such as trails with inclines, declines, and uneven surfaces, adds an element of challenge that further enhances flexibility and balance. These natural obstacles require your muscles and joints to adapt to different movements, promoting overall flexibility and functional strength.

The Role of Walking in Rehabilitation and Injury Prevention

Beyond its benefits for the general population, walking plays a crucial role in rehabilitation and injury prevention. Here's how walking contributes to these areas:

Rehabilitation: For individuals recovering from certain injuries or surgeries, walking is often recommended as part of their rehabilitation program. It provides a low-impact way to restore mobility, strengthen muscles, and improve circulation without putting excessive stress on injured tissues.

Injury Prevention: Regular walking can help prevent injuries by strengthening muscles, improving flexibility, and enhancing overall fitness. Stronger muscles and flexible joints are less prone to strains, sprains, and other musculoskeletal injuries, especially during activities that require physical exertion or repetitive movements.

Incorporating Walking into Your Fitness Routine

Whether you're new to exercise or already engaged in other forms of physical activity, incorporating walking into your fitness routine can offer significant benefits. Here are some tips to make the most of walking for strength and flexibility:

Set Goals: Determine your walking goals, whether it's a certain number of steps per day, a target distance, or a specific duration of walking sessions. Setting achievable goals can keep you motivated and track your progress over time.

Gradual Progression: Start at a comfortable pace and gradually increase the intensity and duration of your walks. This allows your muscles and joints to adapt gradually, reducing the risk of overuse injuries.

Variety: Explore different walking routes and terrains to keep your workouts interesting and challenge your body in new ways. Walking uphill, on trails, or incorporating interval walking (alternating between brisk walking and slower pace) can add variety and enhance the effectiveness of your workouts.

Include Strength Exercises: Combine walking with strength exercises, such as bodyweight exercises, resistance band workouts, or light weight training, to further enhance muscle strength and overall fitness.

Warm-Up and Cool Down: Prior to walking, perform a brief warm-up that includes dynamic stretches to prepare your muscles and joints. After walking, cool down with static stretches to improve flexibility and prevent muscle tightness.

Listen to Your Body: Pay attention to any discomfort or signs of fatigue during walking. Adjust your pace, rest when needed, and consult a healthcare professional if you experience persistent pain or discomfort.

Walking is not just a simple activity; it's a powerful tool for improving strength, flexibility, and overall fitness. By incorporating regular walking into your routine and adopting healthy habits, you can reap the physical, mental, and emotional benefits that walking offers.

Chapter Thirteen
Walking to Overcome Life's Challenges

"Walking through Life's Challenges: Finding Strength, Resilience, and Purpose on the Path"

Life is a journey filled with ups and downs, challenges, and triumphs. At times, it can feel like navigating a winding path with unexpected obstacles along the way. In these moments of difficulty and uncertainty, one of the most powerful tools we have is walking. Walking not only benefits our physical health but also nourishes our mental and emotional well-being, providing a pathway to resilience, strength, and purpose.

The Power of Movement

Walking is a fundamental human activity, deeply ingrained in our nature. It is a simple yet profound act that connects us with our surroundings and with ourselves. When facing life's challenges, whether they are personal, professional, or societal, walking offers a sanctuary where we can pause, reflect, and find solace.

Emotional Healing

Walking also plays a crucial role in emotional healing. It provides a safe space to process emotions, express creativity, and find inner peace. During difficult times, such as loss, grief, or major life changes, walking can be a form of self-care and self-expression. It allows us to connect with our emotions, release pent-up feelings, and move forward with renewed strength and clarity.

Building Resilience

One of the key benefits of walking through life's challenges is the resilience it builds. Walking teaches us perseverance, determination, and adaptability. Every step taken is a testament to our ability to overcome obstacles and keep moving forward. Whether it's a short stroll in nature or a long-distance hike, each walk reinforces our resilience and empowers us to face whatever challenges life throws our way.

Finding Purpose

Walking can also help us find purpose and meaning in difficult times. It allows us to reconnect with our values, passions, and goals. Through contemplative walking practices such as mindfulness walks or walking meditation, we can gain clarity about our priorities and make meaningful choices aligned with our purpose. Walking becomes not just a physical activity but a spiritual journey of self-discovery and growth.

Community Support

In addition to its individual benefits, walking through life's challenges can be enhanced by community support. Joining walking groups, participating in charity walks, or simply walking with friends and family can provide a sense of belonging and solidarity. Sharing experiences, lending a listening ear, and offering encouragement can make the journey through challenges more manageable and meaningful.

Stories of Inspiration

Countless stories of individuals walking through life's challenges inspire us with their resilience, courage, and determination. From survivors of illness and adversity to advocates for social change, walking has been a catalyst for transformation and empowerment. These stories remind us that no matter how difficult the path may seem, walking can lead us to a brighter future filled with hope and possibility.

Walking through life's challenges is not just about putting one foot in front of the other. It's about embracing the journey with courage, resilience, and purpose. By harnessing the power of movement, mindfulness, and community support, we can navigate life's ups and downs with grace and strength. Walking becomes not just a physical activity but a profound metaphor for facing challenges, finding inner strength, and walking toward a brighter tomorrow.

Chapter Fourteen
Walking for Focus and Clarity

Walking is often seen as a physical activity, beneficial for health and fitness. However, its mental and cognitive benefits are equally profound. In this article, we delve into the art of walking for focus and clarity, exploring how this simple yet powerful activity can sharpen your mind, enhance creativity, and improve overall mental well-being.

The Cognitive Science of Walking

To understand why walking is so effective for mental clarity, we must first look at the science behind it. Research has shown that physical activity, including walking, stimulates the release of neurotransmitters such as dopamine and serotonin, which are crucial for mood regulation and cognitive function. Additionally, walking promotes increased blood flow to the brain, delivering oxygen and nutrients that support optimal brain function.

Enhancing Focus through Walking:

One of the key benefits of walking for focus is its ability to break up prolonged periods of sitting and mental exertion. Taking short walking breaks throughout the day can prevent mental fatigue and improve concentration. Moreover, walking in natural environments, such as parks or green spaces, has been shown to have a restorative effect on attention and focus.

Walking Meditation and Mindfulness:

Walking can also be a form of meditation, known as walking meditation or mindful walking. This practice involves paying attention to each step, the rhythm of your breath, and the sensations in your body as you walk. By focusing on the present moment, walking meditation cultivates mindfulness, reduces stress, and enhances cognitive clarity.

Creative Insights on the Move:

Many creative individuals swear by the power of walking to generate ideas and overcoming creative blocks. Walking stimulates divergent thinking, allowing your mind to wander and make unexpected connections. It creates a conducive environment for creative insights to emerge, free from the constraints of a desk or a screen.

The Role of Environment:

The environment in which you walk can significantly impact your mental state and clarity.

Urban walks amidst bustling streets may provide a sense of energy and inspiration, while peaceful nature walks can offer tranquility and a quiet space for reflection. Experimenting with different walking environments can help you find what works best for your focus and clarity.

Incorporating Walking into Daily Routine

Integrating walking into your daily routine doesn't have to be complicated. Simple strategies such as walking meetings, taking phone calls while walking, or scheduling regular walking breaks can make a significant difference in your mental clarity and productivity. Setting aside dedicated time for mindful walks or creative strolls can also enhance the benefits.

Walking for Emotional Well-being:

Beyond cognitive benefits, walking can have a profound impact on emotional well-being. Physical activity, including walking, triggers the release of endorphins, the body's natural feel-good chemicals. This can help alleviate stress, anxiety, and depression, creating a more balanced and focused mind.

Tips for Effective Walking for Focus and Clarity

> ➤ Choose comfortable footwear and attire to make your walks enjoyable.
> ➤ Experiment with different walking speeds and rhythms to see what suits you best.
> ➤ Incorporate mindfulness techniques such as deep breathing or body scans during your walks.

Use walking as an opportunity to unplug from digital distractions and connect with your surroundings.

> ➤ Stay hydrated and nourished to support optimal brain function during walks.

Walking is not just about putting one foot in front of the other; it's a powerful tool for enhancing focus, clarity, and overall well-being. Whether you're seeking a mental refresh, creative inspiration, or a break from the demands of daily life, stepping out for a walk can work wonders for your mind. Embrace the art of walking and experience the transformative benefits it can bring to your cognitive and emotional health.

Opportunity to unplug. When we step away from our screens and endless to-do lists to take a walk, we give our minds much-needed respite. We can use the time to reflect, daydream, observe our surroundings, and reconnect with ourselves. This mental downtime is essential for recharging our focus.

To gain the focus and clarity benefits of walking, try to incorporate it into your daily routine. You don't need to walk for hours - even a 20–30-minute walk can provide a mental boost. If possible, walk in a natural setting like a park or trail, as exposure to green environments enhances cognitive benefits. Unplug from devices and give your mind free rein to wander and reflect.

Over time, regular walking practice can train your brain to drop into a focused state more readily. The next time you're feeling scattered, stuck, or in need of mental refreshment, lace up your shoes and head out for a walk. Take a deep breath, find your stride, and let walking work its magic on your mind. With consistent practice, you may find yourself thinking more clearly, focusing more easily, and tapping into new veins of creativity. In a world of constant distraction, walking can be a simple and powerful way to reclaim your focus and find clarity.

Chapter Fifteen
Walking to Boost Mood and Energy

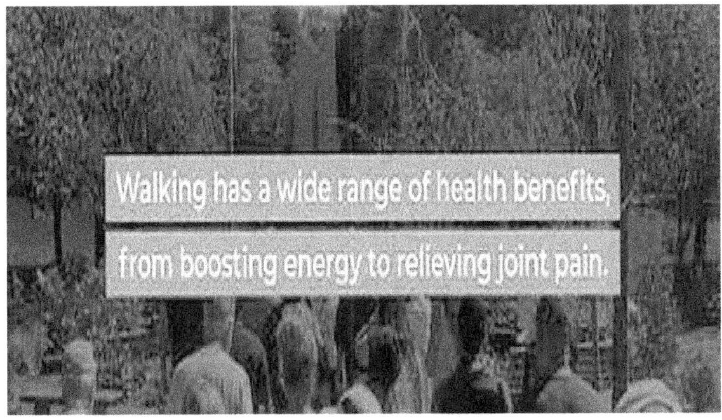

Walking is not only a simple and accessible form of physical exercise but also a powerful tool for improving your mental well-being. In this chapter, we will explore how incorporating walking into your daily routine can significantly boost your mood and energy levels, leading to a happier and more fulfilling life.

The Science Behind Walking and Mood:

Studies have shown that regular walking can have a profound impact on your mental health. When you walk, your body releases endorphins, which are natural mood-enhancing chemicals in the brain. These endorphins interact with receptors in your brain, reducing your perception of pain and triggering positive feelings, like the effects of morphine.

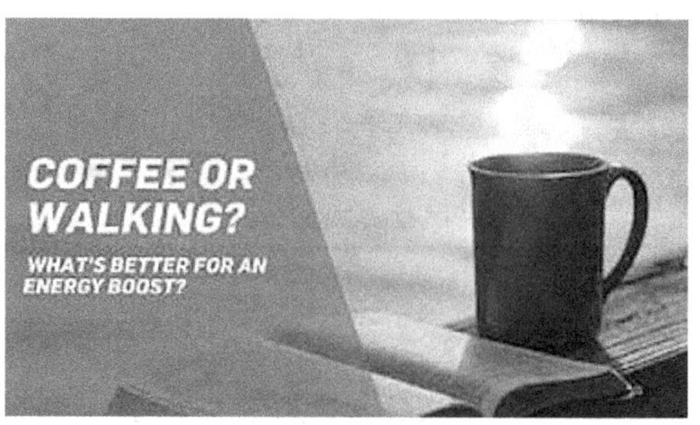

Moreover, walking has been found to reduce levels of cortisol, the stress hormone, in your body. By lowering stress and anxiety, walking can help you feel more relaxed, focused, and emotionally balanced.

Walking and Depression:

Research has demonstrated that walking can be an effective tool in combating depression. In fact, some studies suggest that walking can be as effective as antidepressant medication in treating mild to moderate depression. Regular walking can help alleviate symptoms of depression by promoting the release of neurotransmitters such as serotonin, dopamine, and norepinephrine, which play a crucial role in regulating mood.

Walking and Self-Esteem:

Engaging in regular walking can also contribute to improved self-esteem and self-confidence. As you set and achieve walking goals, you develop a sense of accomplishment and pride in your progress. This can lead to a more positive self-image and increased confidence in your abilities, which can spill over into other areas of your life.

Walking and Energy Levels:

In addition to boosting your mood, walking can also increase your energy levels. When you walk, you improve your circulation, which helps deliver oxygen and nutrients to your cells more efficiently. This, in turn, can help combat feelings of fatigue and sluggishness.

Moreover, walking can help regulate your sleep-wake cycle. By engaging in regular physical activity during the day, you can improve the quality of your sleep at night, leading to more restful and rejuvenating sleep. Better sleep translates to increased energy levels during the day.

Incorporating Walking into Your Daily Routine:

To reap the mood and energy-boosting benefits of walking, aim to incorporate it into your daily routine. Start with short, manageable walks and gradually increase the duration and intensity as you build endurance. Consider walking during your lunch break, taking the stairs instead of the elevator, or going for a brisk walk in the evening after dinner.

Remember, consistency is key. Aim for at least 30 minutes of walking most days of the week to experience the full range of mental health benefits.

Stories of Inspiration

Countless stories of individuals walking through life's challenges inspire us with their resilience, courage, and determination. From survivors of illness and adversity to advocates for social change, walking has been a catalyst for transformation and empowerment. These stories remind us that no matter how difficult the path may seem, walking can lead us to a brighter future filled with hope and possibility.

Walking through life's challenges is not just about putting one foot in front of the other. It's about embracing the journey with courage, resilience, and purpose. By harnessing the power of movement, mindfulness, and community support, we can navigate life's ups and downs with grace and strength. Walking becomes not just a physical activity but a profound metaphor for facing challenges, finding inner strength, and walking toward a brighter tomorrow.

Chapter Sixteen
Walking Your Way to Sleep

Evening Strolls

In today's fast-paced world, sleep has become a precious commodity. Many people struggle with insomnia or poor sleep quality, leading to various health issues and decreased productivity. While there are numerous remedies and strategies to improve sleep, one simple yet highly effective solution often gets overlooked – that is walking. In this chapter, we'll explore the benefits of walking for sleep and how incorporating evening strolls into your routine can transform your nights.

The Sleep Dilemma

Before delving into the role of walking, it's essential to understand why sleep can be elusive for many. Modern lifestyles are characterized by constant stimulation, screen time, and high stress levels, all of which can disrupt our natural sleep patterns. The blue light emitted by electronic devices interferes with melatonin production, the hormone that regulates sleep-wake cycles. Additionally, stress and anxiety can keep our minds racing, making it difficult to unwind and fall asleep.

The Science of Walking and Sleep

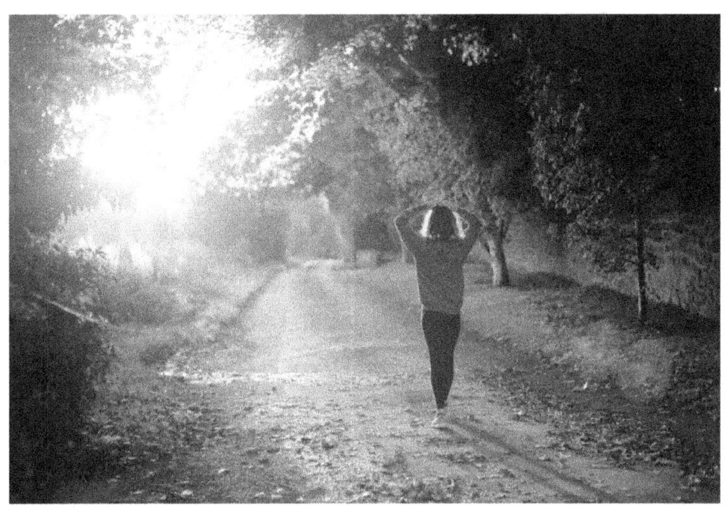

A Brisk Walk Will Help You Sleep Better

Walking, especially in the evening, can significantly impact sleep quality due to several physiological and psychological factors:

Stress Reduction: Walking is a natural stress reliever. It triggers the release of endorphins, often referred to as "feel-good" hormones, which help reduce anxiety and promote relaxation.

Body Temperature Regulation: Physical activity like walking raises body temperature, and as your body cools down after the walk, it mimics the natural drop in temperature that occurs before sleep. This drop in temperature signals to your body that it's time to rest, facilitating a smoother transition to sleep.

Circadian Rhythm Alignment: Regular evening walks help synchronize your internal body clock, known as the circadian rhythm, with the natural cycle of day and night. This alignment can lead to more consistent and restful sleep patterns.

Mindfulness and Relaxation: Walking in nature or peaceful surroundings encourages mindfulness and relaxation. Paying attention to your surroundings, breathing deeply, and focusing on the present moment can calm an overactive mind and prepare it for sleep.

Tips for Walking Your Way to Better Sleep

To maximize the benefits of walking for sleep, consider the following tips:

Timing: Aim for a brisk walk in the early evening, ideally a few hours before bedtime. This allows your body time to cool down and unwind before sleep.

Environment: Choose a quiet, peaceful route for your walk, preferably in natural surroundings like parks or tree-lined streets. The calming effect of nature enhances the relaxation benefits of walking.

Consistency: Make evening walks a regular part of your routine. Consistency reinforces the circadian rhythm and signals to your body that it's time to wind down.

Mindful Walking: Practice mindfulness during your walks by focusing on your breath, senses, and surroundings. Avoid distractions like phones or intense conversations, allowing yourself to fully engage in the experience.

Light Exposure: If possible, walk in natural light or dimly lit environments in the evening. Exposure to natural light during the day and reduced exposure to artificial light at night support healthy sleep-wake cycles.

Post-Walk Routine: After your walk, follow a calming evening routine that promotes relaxation, such as gentle stretching, reading a book, or taking a warm bath. This further prepares your body and mind for a restful night's sleep.

Walking your way to sleep is a powerful yet often overlooked strategy for improving sleep quality. By incorporating evening walks into your routine and following best practices for timing, environment, and mindfulness, you can harness the therapeutic benefits of walking to promote relaxation, align your circadian rhythm, and enjoy more restorative sleep. Embrace the simplicity and effectiveness of this natural remedy and let your evening strolls pave the way to peaceful nights and refreshed mornings.

Chapter Seventeen
Walking for Vitality

Walking, often overlooked in the realm of vigorous exercise, holds a profound key to unlocking longevity and vitality. While high-intensity workouts have their place, the simplicity and accessibility of walking make it a timeless practice that can significantly impact your overall health and well-being. In this article, we delve into the science behind walking and its profound benefits for longevity and vitality.

The Science of Walking

At its core, walking is a natural human movement that engages various muscles and body systems. Research has consistently shown that regular walking can lead to improvements in cardiovascular health, reduced risk of chronic diseases, and enhanced mental well-being. One of the key factors contributing to these benefits is the rhythmic, low-impact nature of walking, which allows individuals of all ages and fitness levels to participate.

Strategies for Walking for Vitality

To harness the full potential of walking for vitality, consider incorporating the following strategies into your routine:

1. Set Realistic Goals

Start with achievable goals that fit your current fitness level and schedule. Gradually increase the duration and intensity of your walks as your stamina improves.

2. Prioritize Consistency

Consistency is key to reaping the benefits of walking. Aim for regular, daily walks or schedule several longer walks throughout the week to maintain momentum and progress.

3. Mix Up Your Routes

Exploring different walking routes keeps your routine interesting and allows you to experience diverse environments. Whether it's urban streets, scenic trails, or park pathways, variety adds to the enjoyment of walking.

4. Focus on Posture and Form

Maintain proper posture while walking to prevent strain and maximize efficiency. Keep your head up, shoulders relaxed, and engage your core muscles for stability.

5. Incorporate Interval Training

Introduce intervals of higher intensity walking or add brief periods of jogging to challenge your cardiovascular system and boost calorie burn.

6. Stay Hydrated and Nourished

Hydration and nutrition play a crucial role in supporting your walking endeavors. Drink plenty of water before, during, and after walks, and fuel your body with balanced meals rich in nutrients.

7. Listen to Your Body

Pay attention to how your body responds to walking. Take breaks when needed, address any discomfort or pain promptly, and adjust your pace or intensity accordingly.

8. Enjoy the Journey

Embrace walking as more than just exercise. Use it as an opportunity to connect with nature, clear your mind, and appreciate the present moment. Find joy in each step you take.

Walking is not merely a means of transportation; it's a powerful pathway to vitality. By embracing walking as a regular practice and incorporating strategies to optimize its benefits, you can enhance your cardiovascular health, prevent chronic diseases, boost your mood, and cultivate a sense of well-being that extends far beyond physical fitness. Start walking today and embark on a journey toward a longer, healthier, and more vibrant life.

Chapter Eighteen
Walking the Happiness Trail

Walking has long been recognized as a simple yet powerful way to boost happiness and well-being. Whether you stroll through nature trails, wander the bustling streets of a city, or enjoy a leisurely walk in your neighborhood, the benefits of walking extend far beyond physical fitness. In this article, we explore why walking is often referred to as the "Happiness Trail" and how it can positively impact your mood, mental health, and overall quality of life.

The Connection Between Walking and Happiness

Endorphin Release: When you walk, your body releases endorphins, also known as the "feel-good" hormones. These chemicals interact with receptors in your brain to reduce pain perception and induce feelings of pleasure and euphoria.

Stress Reduction: Walking outdoors, especially in green spaces like parks or forests, has been linked to lower levels of cortisol, the stress hormone. The peaceful surroundings, fresh air, and gentle exercise combine to create a calming effect on the mind.

Mindfulness and Relaxation: Walking promotes mindfulness, allowing you to focus on the present moment and clear your mind of worries and distractions. It's a form of moving meditation that can enhance relaxation and reduce anxiety.

The Psychological Benefits of Walking

Improved Mood: Regular walking is associated with a more positive mood and decreased feelings of depression and anxiety. The rhythmic motion of walking, coupled with the release of endorphins, uplifts your spirits and fosters a sense of well-being.

Enhanced Creativity: Walking has been shown to stimulate creativity and boost cognitive function. Many great thinkers and writers, such as Charles Dickens and Virginia Woolf, were known to take long walks to refresh their minds and spark creative ideas.

Increased Self-Esteem: Engaging in physical activity like walking can improve self-esteem and self-confidence. Accomplishing walking goals, whether it's completing a certain distance or exploring new routes, contributes to a sense of achievement and empowerment.

Walking as a Social and Community Activity

Connecting with Others: Walking can be a social activity that strengthens relationships and fosters a sense of community. Joining walking groups or simply taking walks with friends or family provides opportunities for meaningful conversations and shared experiences.

Support and Encouragement: Being part of a walking community offers support and encouragement, especially during challenging times. Sharing stories, offering advice, and celebrating achievements together create a sense of belonging and camaraderie.

Practical Tips for Walking Happiness

Set Realistic Goals: Start with achievable walking goals based on your fitness level and schedule. Gradually increase the duration or intensity of your walks as you build stamina and confidence.

Explore New Routes: Keep your walks interesting by exploring different routes and environments. Discovering new parks, trails, or neighborhoods adds variety and excitement to your walking routine.

Practice Mindful Walking: Focus on your surroundings, breathe deeply, and tune in to the sensations of walking. Mindful walking enhances the relaxation and mindfulness benefits of walking, making it a holistic experience for body and mind.

Stay Consistent: Make walking a regular part of your routine. Aim for at least 30 minutes of brisk walking most days of the week to experience the full benefits of walking for happiness and well-being.

Walking is not just a physical activity; it's a journey to happiness and holistic well-being. By incorporating walking into your daily life, you can experience the profound effects it has on your mood, mental health, and overall quality of life. Whether you walk solo, with friends, or as part of a community, the "Happiness Trail" awaits, inviting you to step into a brighter, happier future, one step at a time.

Chapter Nineteen
Walking: A Journey of Redemption

For many of us, walking starts out as simply a mode of transportation - a way to get from point A to point B. But over time, as we take more steps and log more miles, walking can transform into something much more profound and meaningful. With each stride, walking gives us the opportunity to not only improve our physical health, but to embark on an internal journey of reflection, growth, and, redemption.

When life becomes challenging and we feel lost, overwhelmed or burdened by mistakes of the past, walking provides a path forward.

Out on the open road or trail, away from the noise and distractions of daily life, we can begin to process difficult emotions, untangle complex problems, and gradually let go of regrets and pain that may have been weighing us down. The steady rhythm of our footsteps and the calming presence of nature act as a form of moving meditation, allowing our minds to relax, wander and work through issues in a gentle way.

As we walk more, we build not only physical endurance but also emotional and mental resilience. Long solo walks become cherished respites that recharge us and provide clarity. We start to crave that time alone with our thoughts and realizations that come with each walk. Gradually, with every mile traveled, we feel lighter, more unburdened, and more at peace. Walking becomes a way to reconnect with our authentic selves and rediscover a sense of purpose and direction.

Over time, walking can be a powerful tool for redemption - a way to make amends, forgive ourselves, release the past, and step forward into a brighter future. Out on our walks, we find we are better able to put things in perspective, see solutions instead of dwelling on problems, and feel motivation to make positive changes. We start to see that we are capable of overcoming challenges and that a new path is always possible, one step at a time.

As we heal and redeem ourselves through walking, we may feel called to walk with others and share the profound gifts we've received. Walking with friends, family or in community becomes a way to deepen connections, support each other's journeys and walk each other home.

We may even discover that our most important walks are not actually our own but those we take in the service of others.

Walking teaches us that redemption is not a destination but an ongoing journey of putting one foot in front of the other, staying true to our path and trusting that with each step, we are moving in the right direction. Walking becomes a form of personal pilgrimage, a sacred time to reconnect with our highest selves and most cherished values. And we learn that by walking through whatever life brings with grace, resilience and an open heart, we will always find our way home.

Chapter Twenty
Walking to a Sharper Mind

We all know that walking provides excellent physical health benefits - it strengthens the heart, improves circulation, builds endurance, and helps maintain a healthy weight. But did you know that walking is also one of the best things you can do for your brain health and cognitive function?

Numerous scientific studies have shown that regular walking, especially as we get older, can help keep the mind sharp and may even lower the risk of age-related memory loss, dementia, and Alzheimer's disease. Walking increases blood flow and oxygen to the brain, which nourishes brain cells and helps the brain operate at peak efficiency. The increased blood flow from walking also encourages the development of new blood vessels and brain cell connections.

In a study of over 1,000 older adults, those who walked more than 72 blocks per week had greater gray matter volume in key brain regions 9 years later compared to those who walked less. Gray matter contains most of the brain's neurons and is involved in memory, emotions, decision-making, and self-control. Walking is especially beneficial for the hippocampus, the brain region involved in verbal memory and learning.

Walking also stimulates the release of beneficial brain chemicals and growth factors that promote the health of brain cells, such as endorphins, BDNF (brain-derived neurotrophic factor), and VEGF (vascular endothelial growth factor). Higher levels of these substances are associated with better memory, mood, and overall brain function. Even short 10-minute walks can provide a mental boost.

In addition to its direct effects on the brain, walking also reduces stress and improves sleep, both of which are important for optimal brain health and clear thinking. Chronic stress floods the brain with cortisol which can impair memory. Sleep deprivation negatively impacts focus, memory consolidation, and problem-solving skills. Walking in nature seems to be especially beneficial for lowering stress and rumination.

In addition to keeping your body healthy, walking is one of the best things you can do to keep your mind sharp as you age. Aim to walk at least 30 minutes most days - your brain will thank you! .

Chapter Twenty-One
"Ruking" – A New Way to Walk

Ruking: The Ultimate Outdoor Fitness Trend

In the world of fitness, there's always a new trend or activity that captures the attention of enthusiasts looking for fresh and exciting ways to stay in shape. One such trend that has been gaining popularity in recent years is "Ruking," a form of walking that offers a unique and challenging outdoor workout experience.

What is Ruking?

Ruking is a hybrid of walking, running, and hiking, where participants traverse varied terrain, including trails, hills, and mountains, at a pace that falls somewhere between a run and a brisk walk. The term "Ruking" is derived from the combination of the words "run" and "hike," accurately describing the nature of the activity.

Unlike traditional running, which often takes place on flat, paved surfaces, Ruking involves navigating uneven terrain, requiring participants to engage a wider range of muscles and develop greater balance and stability. This added challenge not only provides a more comprehensive workout but also keeps the experience engaging and mentally stimulating.

Benefits of Ruking

Full-body workout: Ruking engages multiple muscle groups, including the legs, core, and upper body, as participants navigate challenging terrain and maintain balance. This leads to improved overall strength and endurance.

Cardiovascular health: The sustained elevated heart rate during Ruking sessions helps improve cardiovascular health, reducing the risk of heart disease and other related conditions.

Reduced impact on joints: Compared to running on hard, flat surfaces, Ruking's varied terrain and softer trails put less stress on the joints, making it a more suitable option for those with joint concerns or injuries.

Mental well-being: Exercising in nature has been shown to reduce stress, improve mood, and boost mental clarity. Ruking allows participants to disconnect from the distractions of daily life and immerse themselves in the beauty of the outdoors.

Adaptability: Ruking can be tailored to suit various fitness levels and preferences, with participants choosing trails based on their difficulty and duration. This adaptability makes it an accessible activity for a wide range of people.

Getting Started with Ruking

To begin your Ruking journey, start by finding suitable trails in your area. Many parks, nature reserves, and mountain ranges offer well-maintained trails that cater to different skill levels. It's essential to choose a trail that aligns with your current fitness level and gradually progress to more challenging routes as your strength and endurance improve.

Proper footwear is crucial for Ruking, as the uneven terrain demands adequate support and traction. Invest in a pair of trail running shoes or hiking boots with good grip and ankle support to prevent injuries and ensure a comfortable experience.

It's also important to carry essential supplies, such as water, snacks, a map, and a first-aid kit, especially when exploring unfamiliar or remote trails. Always inform someone of your planned route and expected return time before setting out on your Ruking adventure.

Ruking Communities and Events

As Ruking gains popularity, communities and events centered around the activity have begun to emerge. Joining a local Ruking group can provide a supportive environment, offering encouragement, advice, and the opportunity to explore new trails with like-minded individuals.

Many areas now host organized Ruking events, ranging from casual group runs to competitive races. These events often showcase the most scenic and challenging trails in the region, attracting participants from all walks of life and fitness levels.

The Future of Ruking

As more people discover the benefits and joys of Ruking, the trend is likely to continue growing in popularity. With its combination of physical challenge, mental stimulation, and outdoor immersion, Ruking offers a unique and rewarding fitness experience that appeals to a wide audience.

As the Ruking community expands, we can expect to see more trails being developed and maintained, as well as an increase in organized events and competitions. This growth will not only make Ruking more accessible to newcomers but also foster a sense of camaraderie and shared passion among participants.

Ruking is an exciting and dynamic fitness trend that offers a multitude of benefits for both physical and mental well-being. By combining the best elements of running and hiking, Ruking provides a challenging and engaging workout that can be enjoyed by people of all ages and fitness levels. As the popularity of Ruking continues to rise, there's never been a better time to lace up your trail shoes and hit the trails. So why not give Ruking a try and discover the joy of exploring the great outdoors while getting in the best

Chapter Twenty-Two
Walking Community – Benefits and Bonds

Walking is not just a solo activity; it can also be a deeply communal experience. From organized walking groups to impromptu gatherings of neighbors strolling together, the walking community plays a significant role in enhancing both physical health and social bonds. In this article, we'll explore the benefits of being part of a walking community and how it fosters connections and well-being.

The Power of Community Walking

Walking is often seen as an individual pursuit, but when done in a group or community setting, its benefits multiply. Here are some key advantages:

Motivation and Accountability: Joining a walking group or community provides built-in motivation to stick to a walking routine. Knowing that others are counting on you can significantly increase your commitment to regular exercise.

Social Interaction: Walking with others allows for meaningful social interaction, fostering friendships and reducing feelings of isolation. It's a chance to connect with like-minded individuals who share your interest in health and wellness.

Variety and Exploration: Group walks often involve exploring new routes and areas, adding variety to your walking experience. This can make your walks more enjoyable and help prevent boredom.

Safety: Walking in a group can enhance safety, especially in unfamiliar or dimly lit areas. There's a sense of security in numbers, reducing concerns about personal safety during walks.

Emotional Support: The camaraderie of a walking community provides emotional support during challenging times. Sharing experiences and lending a listening ear can be incredibly comforting.

Building Bonds Through Walking

The bonds formed within a walking community go beyond fitness goals; they create a sense of belonging and shared purpose. Here's how walking strengthens these bonds:

Shared Experiences: Walking together creates shared experiences and memories. Whether it's overcoming a tough trail or enjoying a scenic route, these shared moments strengthen the bond among walkers.

Supportive Environment: Walking communities often foster a supportive environment where members encourage and uplift each other. This positive reinforcement boosts motivation and self-esteem.

Healthy Competition: Friendly competition within a walking group can be motivating. Setting group goals or participating in walking challenges adds a fun element to the experience.

Knowledge Sharing: Walkers in a community often share tips, tricks, and information about walking techniques, gear, and local routes. This exchange of knowledge enhances everyone's walking experience.

Celebrating Milestones: Achieving milestones together, whether it's reaching a certain distance or improving fitness levels, is celebrated within the community. This sense of achievement is amplified when shared with others.

The Impact on Mental Well-Being

Beyond the physical benefits, being part of a walking community positively impacts mental well-being:

Reduced Stress: Walking in a group or with friends can lower stress levels and promote relaxation. The combination of physical activity and social interaction is a powerful stress-relief strategy.

Improved Mood: The endorphins released during exercise, combined with the social support of a walking community, contribute to improved mood and overall happiness.

Sense of Belonging: Belonging to a walking community provides a sense of belonging and connection, which are vital for mental health. It combats feelings of loneliness and enhances emotional resilience.

Mindfulness and Reflection: Walking in nature with others encourages mindfulness and reflection. It's a time to unplug from digital distractions, be present in the moment, and appreciate the beauty around us.

Sense of Purpose: Having regular walking meetups or group activities gives a sense of purpose and structure to one's routine. It adds meaning to everyday activities and promotes a sense of fulfillment.

Tips for Joining or Creating a Walking Community

If you're interested in reaping the benefits of a walking community, here are some tips:

Research Local Groups: Look for walking groups or clubs in your area. Many communities have organized walking events or regular group walks.

Start Small: If you can't find a group that suits your needs, consider starting one yourself. Invite friends, neighbors, or coworkers to join you for walks and gradually expand your community.

Use Technology: Utilize apps or online platforms designed for connecting with walkers in your area. These platforms can help you find walking partners or create virtual walking challenges.

Set Goals: Whether it's a distance goal, a charity walk, or simply committing to regular walks with friends, setting goals adds purpose and motivation to your walking routine.

Be Inclusive: Create a welcoming and inclusive environment in your walking community. Encourage people of all fitness levels and backgrounds to join, promoting diversity and mutual support.

The walking community offers a wealth of benefits, from improved physical health to enhanced social connections and mental well-being. Whether you join an existing group or start your own, walking together creates a sense of camaraderie, support, and shared experiences. Embracing the walking community can transform your walking routine into a fulfilling and enriching journey.

Chapter Twenty-Three
Exploring Nature on Foot

Exploring Nature on Foot: A Journey of Connection and Discovery

In our modern, fast-paced world, filled with technology and constant connectivity, the simple act of walking in nature has become a rare and precious experience. Yet, amidst the hustle and bustle of daily life, there lies a profound opportunity to reconnect with ourselves, and the natural world around us through the age-old practice of walking. In this chapter we will delve into the transformative power of exploring nature on foot, exploring its benefits for physical health, mental well-being, and our connection to the environment.

The Call of the Wild: Rediscovering Nature's Beauty

Walking in nature is more than just a physical activity; it is a holistic experience that engages all our senses. The rustling of leaves, the scent of wildflowers, the feel of the earth beneath our feet – these sensory stimulations awaken a deep sense of connection to the natural world. Research has shown that spending time in nature can reduce stress, anxiety, and depression, promoting a sense of calm and well-being. As we meander through forests, along rivers, and across meadows, we are reminded of the intricate beauty and harmony of the natural world, fostering a profound appreciation for its wonders.

The Health Benefits of Nature Walking

Aside from its mental and emotional benefits, walking in nature offers numerous advantages for physical health. Unlike the repetitive movements of treadmill walking or indoor exercise, walking on uneven terrain engages a wider range of muscles, improving balance, strength, and flexibility. Studies have also highlighted the cardiovascular benefits of hiking and nature walking, with regular outdoor activity linked to lower blood pressure, reduced risk of heart disease, and improved overall fitness levels.

Mindfulness in Motion: Embracing the Present Moment

One of the most significant gifts of exploring nature on foot is the practice of mindfulness. As we step away from the distractions of screens and schedules, we enter a state of heightened awareness, fully present in the moment. Each footfall becomes a meditation, a rhythmic dance with the earth. This mindfulness in motion not only reduces stress but also cultivates a deeper connection to us and our surroundings. Through mindful walking, we learn to appreciate the small wonders – a delicate flower, a hidden stream, the play of light through leaves – fostering a sense of gratitude and wonderment.

Ecotherapy: Healing the Planet and Ourselves

Beyond personal well-being, walking in nature also carries profound implications for environmental stewardship. As we immerse ourselves in natural landscapes, we develop a stronger sense of environmental awareness and responsibility. This ecological mindfulness inspires us to protect and preserve the fragile ecosystems that sustain life on Earth. Many ecotherapy programs utilize nature walking as a therapeutic tool, harnessing the healing power of the outdoors to promote both individual and planetary health.

The Art of Slow Travel: Exploring at Nature's Pace

In a world obsessed with speed and instant gratification, walking offers a refreshing antidote – the art of slow travel. Unlike cars or trains that whisk us from one destination to another, walking allows us to savor the journey itself. It encourages us to take detours, follow winding paths, and discover hidden treasures off the beaten track. This unhurried approach to travel not only deepens our connection to nature but also fosters a sense of adventure and exploration, transforming a simple walk into a transformative odyssey.

Cultivating a Culture of Walking in Nature

As we recognize the myriad benefits of exploring nature on foot, it becomes imperative to cultivate a culture that encourages and supports walking in natural environments. This includes creating accessible trails, preserving green spaces, and promoting outdoor education and recreation. By integrating walking into our daily lives and communities, we can foster a healthier, happier society connected to the rhythms of nature.

Walking as a Path to Renewal and Connection

In conclusion, exploring nature on foot is not just a leisure activity; it is a profound journey of renewal and connection. From the physical benefits of improved fitness and cardiovascular health to the mental and emotional rewards of reduced stress and increased mindfulness, walking in nature offers a holistic approach to well-being. Moreover, it fosters a deep appreciation for the beauty and diversity of our natural world, inspiring us to become better stewards of the Earth. So, lace up your shoes, step outside, and embark on a transformative adventure along nature's trails — for in every step lies a world of discovery and wonder.

Appendix "A"
'Walking'
"Henry David Thoreau"

In his essay Thoreau extols the virtues of immersing oneself in nature and laments the inevitable encroachment of private ownership upon the wilderness.

Walking
By Henry David Thoreau

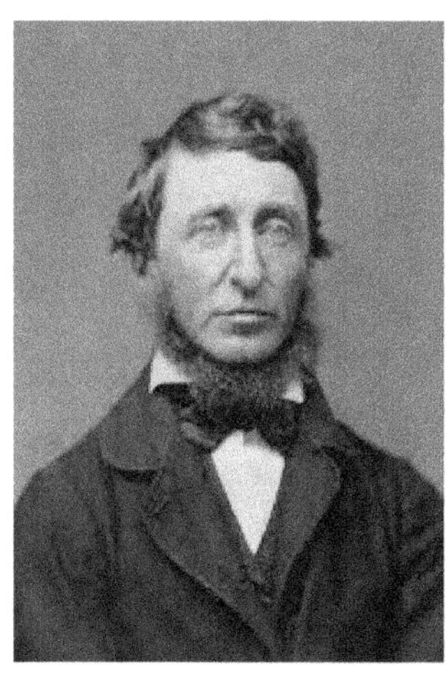

I wish to speak a word for Nature, for absolute freedom and wildness, as contrasted with a freedom and culture merely civil, — to regard man as an inhabitant, or a part and parcel of Nature, rather than a member of society. I wish to make an extreme statement, if so, I may make an emphatic one, for there are enough champions of civilization: the minister and the school committee and every one of you will take care of that.

I have met with but one or two persons in the course of my life who understood the art of Walking, that is, of taking walks, — who had a genius, so to speak, for sauntering: which word is beautifully derived "from idle people who roved about the country, in the Middle Ages, and asked charity, under pretense of going à la Sainte Terre," to the Holy Land, till the children exclaimed, "There goes a Sainte-Terrer," a Saunterer, — a

Holy-Lander. They who never go to the Holy Land in their walks, as they pretend, are indeed mere idlers and vagabonds; but they who do go there are saunterers in the good sense, such as I mean. Some, however, would derive the word from sans terre without land or a home, which, therefore, in the good sense, will mean, having no particular home, but equally at home everywhere. For this is the secret of successful sauntering. He who sits still in a house all the time may be the greatest vagrant of all; but the saunterer, in the good sense, is no more vagrant than the meandering river, which is all the while sedulously seeking the shortest course to the sea. But I prefer the first, which, indeed, is the most probable derivation. For every walk is a sort of crusade, preached by some Peter the Hermit in us, to go forth and reconquer this Holy Land from the hands of the Infidels.

It is true, we are but faint-hearted crusaders, even the walkers, nowadays, who undertake no persevering, never-ending enterprises. Our expeditions are but tours and come round again in the evening to the old hearthside from which we set out. Half the walk is but retracing our steps. We should go forth on the shortest walk, perchance, in the spirit of undying adventure, never to return, — prepared to send back our embalmed hearts only as relics to our desolate kingdoms. If you are ready to leave father and mother, and brother and sister, and wife and child and friends, and never see them again, — if you have paid your debts, and made your will, and settled all your affairs, and are a free man, then you are ready for a walk.

Henry David Thoreau was an essayist, a poet, and a philosopher.

Appendix "B"
The History of Walking

In modern day society where there are technology-driven activities, walking remains a timeless and universal practice. Its simplicity, accessibility, and myriad benefits continue to make it a cherished activity for individuals seeking physical, mental, and emotional well-being.

From the dawn of human evolution to the digital age, walking has woven itself into the fabric of human experience. It has been a mode of survival, a means of exploration, a form of expression, and a path to health and happiness. As we reflect on the history of walking, we recognize not only its enduring importance but also its potential to guide us on a journey of discovery, connection, and fulfillment.

Walking, an activity that seems so natural and effortless to us today, has a rich and fascinating history that stretches back to the earliest days of human existence. From the evolution of bipedalism to the development of walking as a recreational and health-promoting activity, the journey of walking through history is a testament to its enduring significance in human life.

Early Human Walking: The Evolution of Bipedalism

The story of walking begins millions of years ago with the evolution of bipedalism. Our early ancestors, who were once quadrupedal like other primates, gradually transitioned to walking on two legs. This adaptation allowed them to free their hands for tool use and manipulation, marking a pivotal moment in human evolution.

Evidence of bipedalism can be traced back to Australopithecus afarensis, an early hominid species that lived over 3 million years ago. The famous fossilized skeleton known as "Lucy" is a prime example of this transitional form, showcasing the upright posture and bipedal gait characteristic of human walking.

Walking in Ancient Civilizations

As human societies developed and civilizations emerged, walking played a crucial role in daily life. In ancient civilizations such as Mesopotamia, Egypt, Greece, and Rome, walking was not just a means of transportation but also a symbol of status and power.

In ancient Rome, for instance, the concept of the "peripatetic philosopher" emerged, referring to philosophers like Aristotle who engaged in philosophical discussions while walking. This practice not only promoted intellectual stimulation but also highlighted the connection between walking and contemplation.

Walking in Religious and Spiritual Contexts

Many religious and spiritual traditions incorporate walking as a form of devotion, meditation, or pilgrimage. For example, in Buddhism, walking meditation (known as kinhin) is practiced as a complement to seated meditation, emphasizing mindfulness and awareness of each step.

Pilgrimages, such as the Camino de Santiago in Spain or the pilgrimage to Mecca in Islam, involve extensive walking journeys undertaken for spiritual fulfillment and enlightenment. These sacred walks have deep historical roots and continue to attract pilgrims from around the world.

The Rise of Walking as Recreation

During the Renaissance and Enlightenment periods, walking gained popularity as a recreational activity among the upper classes. Prominent figures like Henry David Thoreau and Ralph Waldo Emerson extolled the virtues of walking in nature, advocating for its restorative and inspirational benefits.

In the 19th century, the development of urban parks and public gardens further promoted walking as a leisurely pursuit. The creation of pedestrian-friendly spaces encouraged people to walk for pleasure and health, leading to the emergence of walking clubs and organized walking tours.

Walking for Health and Wellness

The 20th century witnessed a growing recognition of walking's health benefits. Medical professionals began prescribing walking as a form of exercise for improving cardiovascular health, managing weight, and enhancing overall well-being. Walking became accessible to people of all ages and fitness levels, offering a low impact yet effective way to stay active.

The concept of "walkability" also gained prominence in urban planning, with cities striving to create pedestrian-friendly environments that prioritize safety, accessibility, and connectivity. Sidewalks, crosswalks, and pedestrian bridges became essential features of modern urban landscapes, encouraging walking as a mode of transportation.

Walking in the Digital Age

In the 21st century, walking has evolved alongside technological advancements. Fitness trackers and mobile apps have made it easier for people to monitor their walking habits, set goals, and track progress. Virtual walking challenges and online communities have also emerged, fostering a sense of camaraderie and motivation among walkers worldwide.

Despite the rise of sedentary lifestyles and technology-driven activities, walking remains a timeless and universal practice. Its simplicity, accessibility, and myriad benefits continue to make it a cherished activity for individuals seeking physical, mental, and emotional well-being.

From the dawn of human evolution to the digital age, walking has woven itself into the fabric of human experience. It has been a mode of survival, a means of exploration, a form of expression, and a path to health and happiness. As we reflect on the history of walking, we recognize not only its enduring importance but also its potential to guide us on a journey of discovery, connection, and fulfillment.

About the Author

Allen Kelley has self-published 22 non-fiction books, and two works of fiction. These books are available on Amazon.com and other bookseller sites in the US and Europe. He has also written (2) screenplays and has co-produced a documentary film.

His writings focus on the plights of the oppressed and the millions of underprivileged individuals who are on the margins of society.

Unfortunately, these individuals have no way to defend themselves, to fight for their rights or to hear their cries for help.,

Allen's writings shed light on the struggles of all marginalized and abused individuals of the world. Their struggles deserve a voice.

Through his writings, Allen brings forth an awareness of the challenges faced by persons from disadvantaged backgrounds.

Allen also created the "Race Against Hunger" in NYC.

Other publications by the author

Books

➢ Ridin' the Rails

- Addiction: Slaying the Dragon
- RCI Points User Guide
- Love and Danger on the Oregon Trail
- A Rousing Dog Story – Told by a Dog
- Mormonism – The Shocking Untold Story
- In the Kingdom of the Dali Llama
- RCI Weeks User Guide
- Walkin Will Save Your Life
- The Mormon Exodus- from Nauvoo to Salt Lake Valley
- Suicide With Food – An American Tragedy
- The Angel Moroni and the Golden Tablets
- The Christmas Time Epiphanies
- Life Begins at 70
- Tibet as it Was - A Photo Journey
- Self-Discovery – Reinvent Yourself for Greater Happiness and Success
- Your Epiphany Awaits

Screenplays

Cowboy Magic – (Treatment Available – filming of the first two scenes under way). Script registered with WGA west

Six Women West – Based the Novel "Love and Danger on the Oregon Trail"

"The Revenge of Apache Warrior Lozen"

Notes

178

Notes

Notes

Notes

Notes

Notes

Notes

184